Interventional Breast Procedures

Cherie M. Kuzmiak

Editor

Interventional Breast Procedures

A Practical Approach

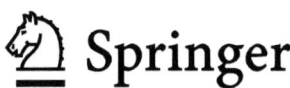 Springer

Editor
Cherie M. Kuzmiak
Department of Radiology
University of North Carolina at Chapel Hill
Chapel Hill, NC
USA

ISBN 978-3-030-13401-3   ISBN 978-3-030-13402-0   (eBook)
https://doi.org/10.1007/978-3-030-13402-0

This Springer imprint is published by the registered company Springer Nature Switzerland AG
The registered company address is: Gewerbestrasse 11, 6330 Cham, Switzerland

Preface

The success of a breast cancer program depends not only on the early detection of suspicious lesions but also on the diagnostic performance and appropriate post-biopsy management of percutaneous breast procedures. Image-guided percutaneous needle core biopsies account for approximately 70–90% of the breast biopsies performed annually in the United States, and the majority of these are benign. Image-guided breast procedures have multiple advantages over open surgical biopsies, which include reduced cost, a less invasive nature, fewer complications, and faster patient recovery.

The intent of this textbook is for the education and training of radiologists currently in practice and those physicians in training (fellows, residents, and medical students). It should be used as an educational tool to help develop image-guided interventional breast procedural skills and how to apply them in a clinical setting. The book is unique in that it pertains exclusively to percutaneous image-guided breast procedures with a patient-centered focus. All of the authors are expert radiologists, trained in breast imaging, and are dedicated to patient care and teaching.

The first chapter of the book is dedicated to a patient-centered approach. This is extremely important as we transition the practice of radiology from a volume-based to a value-based imaging care. In addition, each image-guided modality (ultrasound, mammography, and magnetic resonance imaging) will be discussed in a separate chapter. Also included in this book is a chapter focusing on the novel technique of digital breast tomosynthesis-guided procedures. To conclude the book, there is a devoted chapter to radiology and pathology in concordance with lesion management. We hope the readers will find this book both interesting and helpful.

"The whole purpose of education is to turn mirrors into windows." —Sydney J. Harris

Chapel Hill, NC, USA   Cherie M. Kuzmiak

Contents

Contributors

Andrea Arieno, BS Elizabeth Wende Breast Care, LLC, Rochester, NY, USA

Amy S. Campbell AdventHealth Medical Group - Radiology at Central Florida, Orlando, FL, USA

Stamatia Destounis, MD Elizabeth Wende Breast Care, LLC, Rochester, NY, USA

Romuald Ferre, MD Department of Radiology, Montreal General Hospital Site, McGill University, Montreal, QC, Canada

Cherie M. Kuzmiak, DO, FACR, FSBI Department of Radiology, UNC School of Medicine, University of North Carolina, Chapel Hill, NC, USA

Dag Pavic, MD Medical University of South Carolina, Charleston, SC, USA

Amanda Santacroce, BA Elizabeth Wende Breast Care, LLC, Rochester, NY, USA

Jean M. Seely, MDCM, FRCPCM University of Ottawa, Ottawa, ON, Canada
Ottawa Hospital Research Institute, Ottawa, ON, Canada
The Ottawa Hospital, Ottawa, ON, Canada

Mary Scott Soo, MD Duke University Medical Center, Durham, NC, USA

Chapter 1
Interventional Procedures: Patient-Centered Approach

Mary Scott Soo

Introduction

While technical skills and advances in imaging technologies capture much of the radiologist's focus in clinical settings, at times we need a reminder that the patients are at the center of the care we provide; they should matter the most. For decades, breast imaging has been the radiology leader in a patient-centered approach to care, with development of federal requirements (Mammography Quality Standards Act [MQSA]) and the Breast Imaging Reporting and Data System (BI-RADS™) lexicon to guide care [1, 2]. Throughout this process, breast imaging radiologists have directly informed not only providers but also patients of mammography results, and many have engaged in daily face-to-face discussions with patients in their clinics regarding abnormal results and biopsy recommendations [3].

Breast imaging's long-standing dedication to patient communication along with other efforts to enhance patients' experiences has preceded a more recent movement across medicine as a whole, termed patient-centered care (PCC) or patient- and family-centered care [4]. PCC is a form of biopsychosocial care, which treats the patient as a whole person, and has become one of the core values of the Society of Breast Imaging (SBI) [5]. Using this PCC concept, providers ideally collaborate with both patients and families in a shared decision-making process [5, 6]. The patients' needs, goals, and preferences are respected, and treatments encompass not only the physical but also the psychosocial components of illnesses [5–7]. Using the PCC approach to cancer care, physicians are not just sources of information and expertise. They provide emotional support, guidance, and understanding, all of which are enduring characteristics in physician-patient relationships that are valued by cancer patients [7–10].

M. S. Soo (✉)
Duke University Medical Center, Durham, NC, USA
e-mail: Mary.soo@duke.edu

© Springer Nature Switzerland AG 2019
C. M. Kuzmiak (ed.), *Interventional Breast Procedures*,
https://doi.org/10.1007/978-3-030-13402-0_1

PCC serves to improve patient satisfaction, a metric factored into evolving Center for Medicare and Medicaid (CMS) value-based care payment models [8–12]. In an effort to re-evaluate and renew radiology's approach and commitment to patients, a recent nationwide survey found that radiology patients recognize the importance of the imaging examination and radiologists' interpretation; however, they report little interaction with radiologists [13]. This has resulted in a call for activities to increase communication and care coordination in radiology [13, 14]. The American College of Radiology (ACR) through its Imaging 3.0 initiative now provides materials to navigate the newer payment models while enhancing radiologists' awareness and involvement in PCC [15].

Breast imaging has been the model for building radiologist-patient relationships and enhancing care coordination as these initiatives move forward. Many breast-imaging radiologists are quite skilled and compassionate in communications with the anxious patient throughout the biopsy process, quickly developing effective radiologist-patient relationships. Yet they are still willing to make efforts to further improve communication and satisfaction that may be particularly helpful during emotionally stressful breast biopsies [3]. Imaging-guided core-needle breast biopsies are outpatient biopsy procedures performed using local anesthesia, without sedation, to diagnose imaging-detected lesions. Because patients often experience anxiety related to pain during biopsy and uncertainty about a possible cancer diagnosis, evaluating the patient's experience during these breast imaging procedures is the first step in enhancing patient experiences [16]. This chapter will examine patient perspectives of imaging-guided breast biopsy procedures and review important patient-centered interventions and approaches to enhance patient care, particularly related to patient communication, anxiety reduction, reduced wait times, and pain control.

Understanding Patients' Breast Biopsy Experiences

Anxiety Related to a Biopsy Recommendation

Most patients choose to undergo mammography screening because they understand and desire the benefits of early detection and treatment if cancer is detected. However, inherent in undergoing the examination is facing the possibility that breast cancer will actually be detected and the impact this diagnosis could have on the patient's life. The large majority of women receive the good news of a negative mammogram and experience minimal distress in the process. However, for women presenting for diagnostic imaging of a lump or other symptom, or undergoing additional images following a screening study, anxiety develops when they realize that the results may not be normal, and patient anxiety increases as the period of uncertainty progresses [17, 18]. Results in most cases are benign, requiring no further investigation, and often this is communicated to the patient by the technologist performing the exam [3]. Patients with more suspicious abnormalities requiring biopsy will either receive the news from the radiologist during a consultation in the breast imaging clinic following diagnostic imaging or are required to wait much longer until their referring physician contacts them with results [3]. While breast imaging radiologists view this process of diagnosing breast cancer a normal part of their daily work routine, some patients experience the process as one of the greatest challenges of their lives. Reducing delays by incorporating time to effectively communicate biopsy recommendations into breast imaging practices often builds patient connection and trust and enhances satisfaction for the long term [19].

Anxiety can be defined as "a feeling of worry, nervousness, or unease, typically about an imminent event or something with an uncertain outcome" [20]. When presented with a biopsy recommendation, patient anxiety levels vary and manifest in different forms. During the discussions, some patients outwardly appear to accept the news calmly, while others are visibly affected and may experience a variety of emotional responses. These may initially take the form of shock or disbelief, and many experience fear and guilt or project their fear outwardly in the form of anger [7, 21]. A few patients even experience degrees of denial and may refuse to agree to a biopsy [7]. A number of patients report difficulty processing the information because they feel overwhelmed by their beliefs regarding the implications of a potential breast cancer diagnosis, many equating the fear of cancer with the fear of dying [21]. Fear of other potential consequences of breast cancer treatment also enters their thoughts, framed by their family history of cancer and previous exposure to breast cancer patient experiences. Some worry about cancer pain, loss of hair during therapy, and disfigurement from surgery; others fear the financial implications of lost wages or losing control of their lives and connection to others [21, 22]. The level of patient anxiety related to breast biopsies remains clinically significant throughout the biopsy process, and uncertainty of the results remains a strong contributor until results are delivered [16].

Other factors also contribute to patients' anxiety as they progress through the breast biopsy process. In addition to uncertainty about having to face a cancer diagnosis, anticipating the biopsy procedure itself can induce high levels of anxiety. Many patients report being afraid of needles, and the degree of anticipated pain correlates strongly with the degree of pain reported during the biopsy [23]. Beyond procedure-related pain or discomfort, women may worry about taking time off work, arranging care of children or other family members, or worrying family and friends [21, 22].

Waiting for the biopsy is also stressful. For women with low or average levels of chronic life stress, the degree of anxiety increases as wait times for the procedure increase [17]. Many women request same-day biopsies for this reason. Therefore, scheduling the biopsy procedure with as little delay as possible is very beneficial to many women's psychological states. Because of delays caused by the need for orders from referring providers, facility staffing and backlogs, or even the patient's domestic situation, educational counseling about the relative risk of cancer during the biopsy recommendation discussion may be helpful to reduce anxiety, particularly in women with low-risk lesions [24, 25].

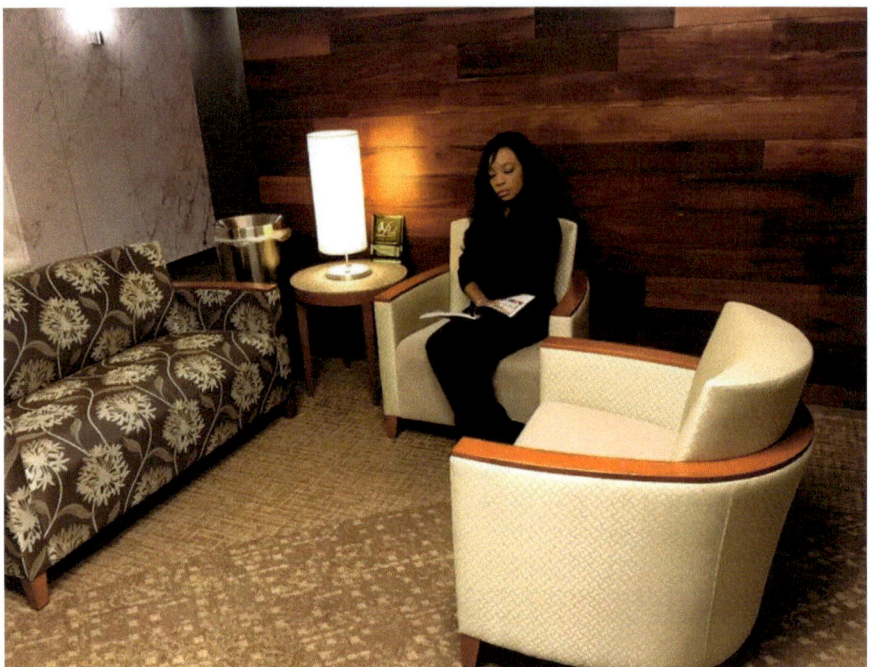

Fig. 1.1 Waiting room with clustered seating that allows adequate privacy and comfort

Other than receiving a cancer diagnosis at the conclusion of the biopsy process, patient anxiety levels are probably highest on the day of biopsy [17]. Therefore patient comfort, amenities, privacy, and distraction in the waiting room may help them cope with their anxiety. Having a spacious, comfortable waiting room with clustered seating (Fig. 1.1) and a private area for patients and families awaiting biopsy is favored over a crowded waiting room with side-by-side chairs.

Pain and Anxiety During Biopsy

While many patients fear that the imaging-guided biopsy will be painful, actual reported pain levels during these outpatient biopsies are quite low. Studies show that the majority of patients find imaging-guided breast biopsy procedures less painful than expected, with significantly lower average biopsy pain levels (e.g., 1.25 on a 0 to 10 scale), compared to average anticipated pain levels (4.4 on a 0 to 10 scale) [23, 26]. Mean pain ratings reported in several study populations ranged on a 0 to 10 scale from 0.81 using sodium bicarbonate to buffer lidocaine anesthesia injections to 4.3 during MRI-guided biopsies [23, 26–29]. Among different imaging modalities, ultrasound-guided biopsies are reported to be least painful, whereas women report stereotactic and MRI-guided biopsies to be more painful [23, 26–28].

Anxiety Awaiting Results

Patients experience fatigue after biopsies are completed [30]. At that point, anxiety levels decrease from pre-biopsy levels but remain clinically significant until the results are delivered, often 1 day to 1 week later [16, 31]. Physiologic distress as the waiting period progresses can actually equal the distress levels of patients who are given a breast cancer diagnosis [31]. The anxiety and distress highlight the need to deliver results to patients as soon as possible. Although earlier studies reported otherwise, recent studies suggest that patients now want to receive results in the fastest way possible, (e.g., by telephone), as opposed to waiting longer for results in person, and find it acceptable to receive results from the radiologist, as opposed to waiting longer to hear from their referring physician [32–34].

When the results are delivered, receiving a breast cancer diagnosis can induce a crisis in patients' lives. As associated with the biopsy recommendation, patients again may experience cognitive distraction and difficulty processing information [35]. While they might not remember important detailed information conveyed during the discussion, patients do vividly remember how they felt during the conversation. In a study of terminal cancer patients, patients distinctly remembered the attitude of physician delivering news of the cancer diagnosis and whether they felt loved and supported and maintained hope or whether they felt alone and abandoned by the physician's lack of connection and inability to face the issue [21]. Therefore, the radiologist's ability to effectively and compassionately deliver a cancer diagnosis may have a lifetime impact on the patient.

Approaches for Optimal Patient-Centered Care During Biopsies

Benefits of Better Patient Communication

A high degree of technical competency and skill in performing imaging-guided biopsies is obviously critical for optimal patient care and will be reviewed in subsequent chapters. Beyond this, effective radiologist-patient communication is probably the most important factor in the patient-centered approach. Efforts to clearly communicate at all stages of the biopsy experience can impact the degree of patient understanding, provide expectations for procedures, describe effectiveness of supportive interventions, and provide support and encouragement at the time of a cancer diagnosis. Acknowledging patients' perspectives of situations, compassionately evaluating and addressing their needs with communication that supports patient autonomy, contributes to enhanced patient satisfaction [36].

Better radiologist-patient communication prior to biopsies also has the potential to impact the patients' views about mammography and their psychological state during the procedure. Patients who report better communication with the radiologist perceive greater benefits and fewer barriers to mammography screening [37]. In addition, Miller et al. showed that effective radiologist-patient communication both at the time of biopsy recommendation and during the biopsy is inversely associated with patient anxiety; patients who perceived better communication with the radiologist reported lower levels of anxiety at the time of biopsy [16]. Moreover, better patient communication positively impacts cancer treatment, patient outcomes, and psychological symptoms through fewer missed appointments and adherence to treatments [9, 10, 38]. Better communication is associated with higher patient satisfaction among older breast cancer patients and could impact medical reimbursements through CMS patient experience surveys evaluating, among other things, physician-patient communication [7–12, 39].

From another perspective, failure to communicate is the most common cause of medical malpractice, and effective and compassionate communication is inversely associated with malpractice claims. In a study of primary care physicians, those with no medical malpractice claims used more statements educating patients about what to expect and the flow of the visit, checked for understanding, laughed and used humor more, solicited patients' opinions, and encouraged patients to talk, spending longer in routine visits [40]. Conversely, Beckman et al. in a study of settled malpractice suits against a large metropolitan medical center found that "the decision to litigate is most often associated with perceived lack of caring and/or collaboration in health care delivery" [41]. In another study, patients rated surgeons identified with higher malpractice litigation history as having higher dominance and lower concern in their voice tones [42]. Finally, Hickson et al. reported that patients pursuing malpractice claims cited that they felt rushed, never received explanations for tests, and were ignored [43].

On the other extreme, an overly empathetic or emotional reaction on the part of the radiologist might not be helpful either. Many breast imaging radiologists are very compassionate in their interactions with patients; however sympathizing and relating too closely with the patient's situation could lead to emotional vulnerability. If the radiologist experiences a strong emotional response (e.g., tears up along with the patient) when delivering bad news, this response could be misinterpreted by the patient to mean that the situation is more dire than it actually is. Radiologists therefore must be grounded in their own emotional stability, while providing appropriate empathy and compassion. Overall, a balance of focus, patience, compassion, and emotional resiliency can help the radiologist most effectively convey information and recognize and address the patient's needs while delivering results.

How to Communicate "Bad News"

Information sharing and relationship building are linked components of physician-patient relationships that influence breast cancer patients' positive experiences of mastery of their illness experience [44]. Therefore, effective patient communication about breast biopsies contains two types of messages [38, 45, 46]. The content message expresses the information that needs to be conveyed (e.g., a biopsy recommendation, information regarding informed consent, results of a breast biopsy) [38, 45, 46]. Written materials can supplement to the verbal message; for example, a written description (handout, pamphlet) of what to expect during the biopsy procedure, along with a description of the time, date, and location of the procedure, can help alleviate uncertainty about the procedure and reiterate details. These materials can help patients adhere to the scheduled procedure, particularly in situations where patient distress could interfere with cognitive processing of verbal information.

In addition to the content message, a relational message is also an important component to these conversations and expresses how individuals view each other and build a relationship through their interactions [38, 45, 46]. In order to establish a relationship, communications need to reflect the ideals incorporated into the patient-centered care model, where shared decision-making incorporates patient needs and goals [47]. Women diagnosed with breast cancer not only need trust in their physician's expertise but need the physician to develop a unique relationship with them and respect their autonomy [36]. Statements in Table 1.1 reflect what patients request during communications with providers [36, 45, 48, 49].

When the radiologist breaks the bad news that the patient needs to undergo biopsy or has been diagnosed with breast cancer, a number of communication models could be used, and most involve a multi-step approach, encapsulated below [7–10, 44–54]. However, before entering the room or picking up the telephone for any encounter, the radiologist should first tune in to his or her own mental and emotional state [54]. The ability to be attentive and perceptive regarding a patient's clinical status and empathetic while exploring patient concerns and emotions is related to the physician's own well-being [8]. If the radiologist has many patients waiting, films to read, technologists and clinicians demanding his/her time, or has his/her own emotional distractions or vulnerability in the moment, these should be brought into awareness. Identifying these distracting thoughts or emotions allows a choice for releasing them and returning to the present moment. Two or three deep breaths before the encounter can help downregulate any physiological hyper-arousal state that might be associated with the distracting thoughts or stressful emotions [55]. Then, with a clear mind, the radiologist can bring his/her attention fully to the patient and the upcoming conversation and allow for effective communication of the

Table 1.1 What patients want during communications with their provider [36, 45, 48, 49]	
	"Talk with me, not at me"
	"Establish a relationship with me"
	"Acknowledge my feelings"
	"Reassure me"
	"Be easy to talk to"
	"Encourage my questions"
	"Explain my results"

necessary information [55]. This approach can help dissipate the emotional vulnerability related to deep empathy for the patient and best prepare him to appropriately address whatever concerns arise from the patient.

The Biopsy Recommendation Encounter

1. Beyond evaluating the radiologist's own mental and emotional well-being, additional preparation for the encounter is needed. Wearing a white coat helps present a professional appearance. Upon entering the room, a smile, making eye contact, an introduction, a handshake, and sitting eye-to-eye with the patient all help to establish immediate rapport (Fig. 1.2) [54]. In these first few focused seconds, the radiologist also assesses the patient's demeanor and body language, observing whether they feel attentive, open, and engaged in the interaction or anxious, worried, angry, or closed off (Fig. 1.3) [56, 57]. Having the patient's spouse, partner, family, or friends present can be helpful to facilitate understanding of the content and can help ensure follow-up and improve the patient's emotional state. It is important to have a follow-up appointment or other information ready for the patient, to have tissues if the patient becomes tearful, and to allow no interruptions during the interaction (Fig. 1.4).

2. In the next step, the radiologist discloses the news or the "content" of the message (e.g., the results of the diagnostic imaging indicate a biopsy is necessary). When recommending a biopsy for low-risk lesions (e.g., BI-RADS 4A), it is helpful to provide context up front, describing that there is a low likelihood of the lesion being cancer. On the other extreme, when discussing a highly suspicious BI-RADS category 5 lesion, the radiologist must discern the patient's desire for and ability to handle information. In this scenario, waiting in order to assess the

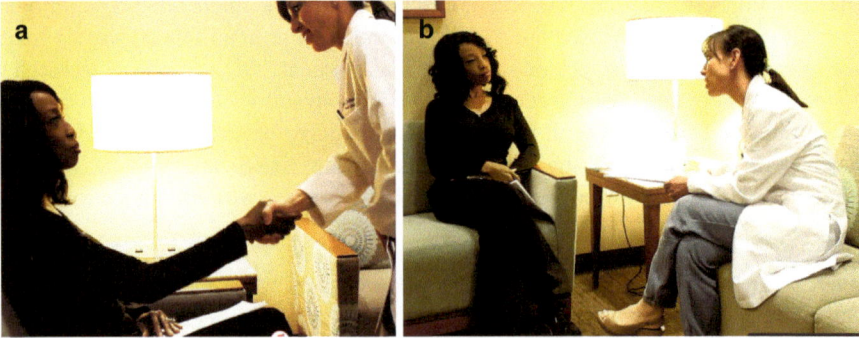

Fig. 1.2 Establishing immediate rapport during biopsy recommendations. (**a**) Upon entering the consultation room, the radiologist wearing a professional-appearing white coat smiles, makes eye contact, and shakes hands with the patient, suggesting warmth, connection, and confidence. (**b**) When discussing the biopsy recommendation, the radiologist is seated eye-to-eye with the patient and leans forward in her seat, a body language that suggests partnership and reliability

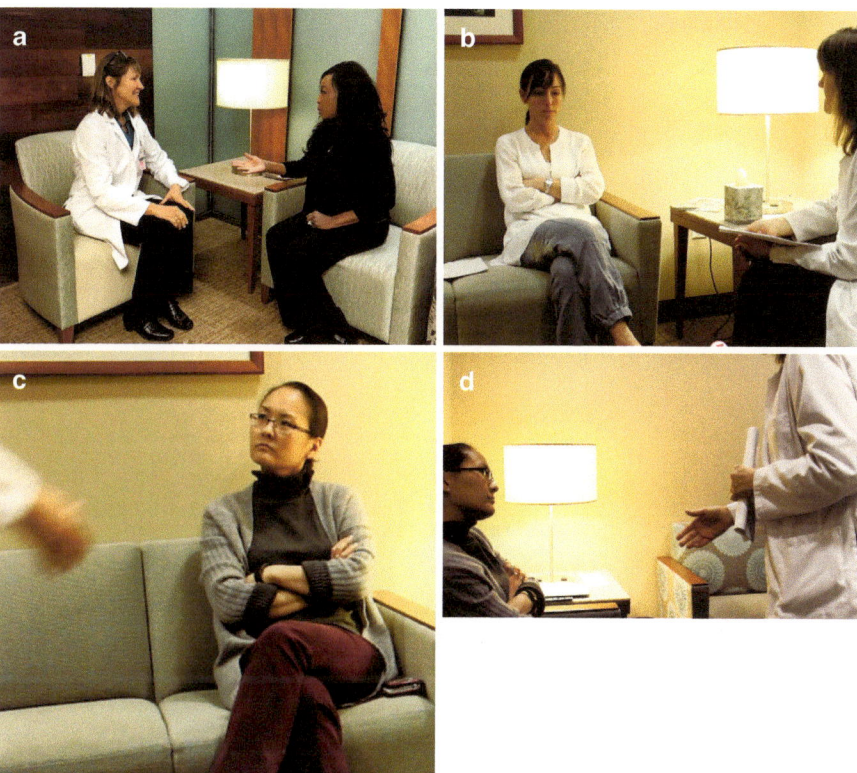

Fig. 1.3 Assessing patients' demeanor and body language. (**a**) During the biopsy recommendation, the patient appears open and engaged in the conversation, leaning forward in her chair, looking the radiologist in the eye, and using hand gesture while communicating. (**b**) The patient in 2b differs from 2a in that she is leaning back in the seat and her legs and arms are crossed, indicating a more closed and distanced posture. She averts her gaze and appears withdrawn, worried, and vulnerable. (**c**) Similar to the patient in 2b, the patient in 2c is also leaning back in her seat with her arms and legs crossed; however, she makes direct eye contact with the radiologist entering the room and has her lips pursed. This appearance relays a closed and more defensive stance. (**d**) The same patient in 2c rejects the radiologist's handshake, maintaining the posture and projecting a guarded, protective, and dissatisfied attitude

patient's initial emotional response to the biopsy recommendation and gauging her desire for information is prudent before describing the high likelihood of cancer. Lay terminology should be used and tailored according to how the radiologist perceives the patient understood the news.

3. After disclosing the news, it is important to pause to evaluate the patient's response. Quietly listening is critical for observing and understanding how the information has been received and processed. The patient may need silence for a short period to let the information sink in, before additional information is presented.

4. The fourth component of the conversation provides additional content, discussing the next steps. Many patients find that having a plan and learning more about

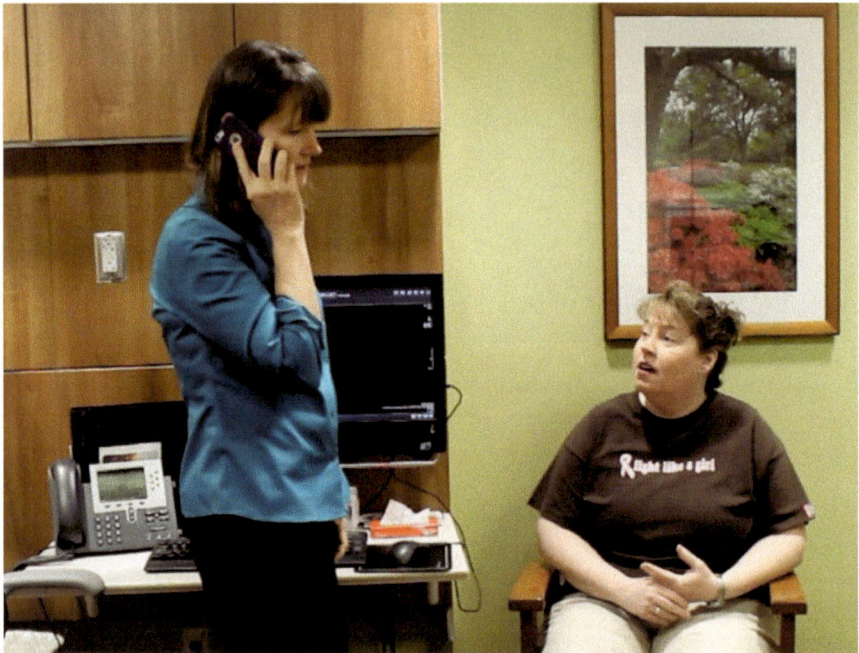

Fig. 1.4 Errors to avoid when communicating biopsy results. Several errors in communication are identified during the illustrated biopsy recommendation encounter. The radiologist is standing above the patient, rather than sitting-eye-to-eye, does not project a professional appearance without a white coat, and allowed an interruption during the conversation by answering her cell phone during the encounter

the upcoming process can help ease the distress of future uncertainty. Having the biopsy appointment ready begins this process and assists in patient adherence to recommended care.

5. After delivering the information, it is important to ensure that the patient understood the information provided. Acknowledging the potential distress from receiving such information, the radiologist should ask the patient to repeat the important take-home points she heard and allow questions to clarify any uncertainties.

6. Finally, offering additional avenues of support can be beneficial. Having references to the American Cancer Society or other related websites can provide additional information. For someone experiencing a strong emotional response to the news, a referral to a cancer care therapist and referring physician may be warranted. Simply asking patients what social support they have and what they might need is a direct way to help manage their care. Providing contact information for questions, a handshake, or even a hug if deemed appropriate can provide emotional support. Ending the conversation warmly and with gratitude concludes the interaction.

Delivering Malignant Biopsy Results

Delivering biopsy results can follow the same multi-step process above; however, some additional specific issues should be considered, particularly when delivering biopsy results by phone [54]. Finding a quiet place for the call without the distractions is important. After contacting the patient and introducing himself/herself, the radiologist should inquire if the patient is in a safe and private place to discuss the biopsy results. Results should not be delivered while the patient is driving. Likewise, she may be at work among colleagues and should be given an opportunity to find a quiet place for the discussion.

Patients often wish to write down the results. It can be helpful at the time of the biopsy procedure to give the patient written materials describing a list of commonly biopsied histological lesions, ranging from benign to malignant. During the subsequent telephone discussion of the results, the radiologist can refer the patient to the specific histological result, numbered under headings of benign, intermediate risk, high risk, or cancer [54]. Additionally, having surgical and other oncology appointments ready when a cancer diagnosis is delivered can assist in patient adherence to recommended care.

When delivering the news by phone, the radiologist does not have the opportunity to read facial expressions and body language, therefore it is important to tune in to verbal clues, and check for clear understanding at the conclusion of the discussion [54]. Describing the result as "positive" or "negative" should be avoided. Patients might interpret a "positive" biopsy to be free of cancer, when the radiologist actually intended to convey the opposite information [54]. Using a phrase such as "Unfortunately, the biopsy specimen did contain cancer cells" is often better received than a phrase such as "You have cancer," which equates the patient herself with a cancer diagnosis [54].

Encouraging patients as they begin their breast cancer healing journey can help empower them in their process. Communications from physicians and others that emphasize rather than minimized the personal significance of the patient's breast cancer experience can promote positive emotional changes regarding quality of life and increased empathy for others [58, 59]. Reflecting on their courage and ability to manage their illness can begin during the breast biopsy experience, as radiologists initiate breast cancer care.

Managing Challenging Scenarios

Emotional Response

If the patient becomes emotional (e.g., tearful), it is not necessary to try to divert or suppress her feelings by presenting more information, conversation, or distraction [54]. These feelings are normal and common among patients receiving bad news.

Quietly allowing her tears is appropriate. The wave of emotion is often short-lived, and the patient may even apologize for the behavior. Acknowledging and understanding that the news is upsetting and that her feelings are normal is the radiologist's appropriate response [54]. This can ease the patient's distress and help her begin to process her grief.

One challenging patient question may be, "Am I going to die of breast cancer?" Acknowledging that many women are concerned with the same question when faced with a breast cancer diagnosis is an appropriate initial reply. Subsequent responses can be adapted depending on the lesion. For a small, localized cluster of calcifications, diagnosed as ductal carcinoma in situ, providing data on the very high survival rates and encouraging the patient to adhere to treatment regimens for optimal outcomes would be appropriate. For others with very aggressive appearing, locally advanced or inflammatory cancers, perhaps with axillary metastases, the radiologist might initially fear that the patient could eventually succumb to the disease. However, the radiologist at that point rarely has all the information or even the expertise to inform the treatment and prognosis in the particular patient's case. Further, he/she should realize that regardless of prognosis, no one at that time-point can actually know the future outcome of the particular individual. Even if statistics would indicate a low percentage 5-year survival, this particular patient could become a remarkable survivor who greatly outlives her prognosis. This information can help reframe the radiologist's outlook. Appropriate comments that are informational, hopeful, and encouraging would include (1) assuring the patient that she will be referred to expert breast oncologists to determine staging, discuss prognosis, and provide treatments, (2) describing improvements in therapies and survival over the years, and (3) encouraging self-care and engagement in her upcoming treatment.

Angry Responses

Occasionally a patient exhibits an angry response at some point during the interactions that could challenge the developing radiologist-patient relationship. Most times, the patient's anger is not directed personally toward the radiologist but may be due to any number of factors creating the patient's current experience. Listening to the patient's concerns without defensiveness or reactivity is paramount at this time to gain trust and rebuild the relationship [54]. Statements in response to these comments that may help the patient feel that their concerns have been heard and might aid in service recovery are suggested in Table 1.2 [45, 54].

Table 1.2 Service recovery statements in response dissatisfaction expressed by the patient [45]

"You seem upset and I am sorry you feel this way. Please tell me more"
"Your feedback is very important to me; our goal is to meet or exceed your expectations and I understand we have not done that"
"I'm sorry we have disappointed you and on behalf of our staff, please accept my apology"
"What can I do to help you right now?"

Table 1.3 Redirecting the conversation [45]

"That's really helpful, thank you. May I now ask a few specific questions?"
"What you've shared with me has given me a more accurate understanding. Thank you"
"That's really helpful, thank you. May I now ask a few specific questions?"
"What you've shared with me has given me a more accurate understanding. Thank you"
"Thank you for sharing these medical concerns. From what I can tell, I don't think they have an impact on your breast abnormality"
"Thank you, that's helpful. Now, I'd like to be sure we review your upcoming biopsy and any questions you may have for me about it"

Redirecting Gracefully for Time Management

The time spent discussing biopsy recommendations or results can range from a few minutes to much longer, depending on the patient and her concerns. Certainly, the radiologist's time for these discussions is limited, and sometimes the conversation needs to be redirected. It is important to realize that patients perceive time more in terms of connection rather than the actual amount of time spent [45, 60]. Therefore, during these discussions, radiologists would add value to the relationship by trying to not speak too quickly so they will not be perceived as rushed [45, 60]. Skillful phrases to help gracefully redirect the conversation are listed in Table 1.3 [45].

Communication and Other Approaches to Enhance Biopsy Procedure Experience

Before the biopsy encounter, the radiologist should review the patient's films and medical record, considering factors that might influence the patient's experience, and evaluate his own state of mind. Upon entering the room, the radiologist can identify clues from the patient's facial expressions and body language about her emotional state, as he establishes rapport, describes the procedure, and obtains informed consent. Patient anxiety and anticipatory pain often predict a more painful patient experience during biopsy [23]; therefore identifying these emotions and addressing them, even briefly, can be helpful and prompt questions to address worrisome issues. "Do you have concerns about undergoing the procedure?" is a simple way to begin the discussion. Perhaps the patient had undergone a previous biopsy experience that proved challenging; if so, acknowledging their concerns or potential for discomfort is important. Determining what was the most difficult part of a previous procedure (e.g., pain, positioning [neck pain, back pain, compression], anxiety about results) can prompt conversation about interventions (e.g., providing more local anesthetic, bolstering positioning to improve patient comfort) to improve the current experience and alleviate anxiety. If pain is the greatest concern, describing that women frequently anticipate higher pain but actually report much lower biopsy pain helps to reassure the patient and may reduce her catastrophic thoughts and perhaps even procedural pain [23]. Emphasizing that the radiologist and biopsy team care about her comfort and will provide adequate and even additional local anesthesia if needed improves patient perceptions of pain control, enhances communication, and helps to build a more trusting radiologist-patient relationship that can improve the overall experience. Patient satisfaction has been shown to correlate more with the perception that caregivers did everything they could to control pain, rather than the actual pain control [61]. They recognize that the team cares about them.

Identifying additional factors that might alleviate the patient's anxiety can also improve the patient's comfort. At times patients with more severe anxiety might request having a family member in the room for support [54, 62]. If this is acceptable to the radiologist and biopsy team, then setting ground rules for safety of the family member is necessary. Having the family member sit in a chair near the foot of the table without a view of the actual procedure field may avoid an unexpected vasovagal reaction that could occur if the family member were to stand next to the patient and watch the procedure [54, 62].

Some patients request prayer with their physician before medical procedures. This has engendered controversy in the minds of providers for many years and may feel unsettling to the radiologist or breast biopsy team, particularly if spiritual or religious beliefs differ between the patient and medical team [63, 64]. However, prayer may be a strong support for patients challenged by serious medical problems [65]. As a component of patient-centered care, addressing patients' requests for prayer at the time of breast biopsies could provide needed support and build the patient-physician relationship [63]. If the patient offers clues or directly asks to pray with the radiologist prior to the procedure, exploring the patient's concerns could guide the conversation [63]. This could be a request for human connection that an empathetic response might satisfy, or for spiritual support based on religious beliefs [63]. Listening and responding respectfully are important. As summarized in Table 1.4. Christensen et al. reviewed this process and potential responses to

Table 1.4 Potential responses to patient requests for prayer [62]

1. "I understand it is important for you to have support at this time. Tell me more"
2. "I hear that you are worried about the biopsy being painful, and that your faith is a source of strength for you. I will keep you in my thoughts and do everything I can to make you comfortable"
3. "I understand that you are worried about results of the biopsy, and that your faith is an important source of strength for you. Let's spend a few moments of silence together"
4. "I understand that prayer is very important to you and I am very willing to stay with you while you pray"
5. If the radiologist is asked if he prays but uncomfortable discussing his faith, a reply could be "I am uncomfortable discussing my faith, however I am more than willing to be here with you while you pray"
6. "I understand this is scary for you. I am glad to silently pray with you"
7. "I understand this is scary for you. Please lead us in prayer"

requests for prayer, based on the physician's personal decisions and views about prayer [63]. These responses could support the patient-physician relationship by allowing physicians to remain present with the patient but also staying true to their own beliefs [63, 64]. If the radiologist agrees to lead the prayer, asking in general for support during the biopsy and ease of fear in the time of uncertainty rather than for specific outcomes would be the most appropriate, given potential for differences in beliefs about the purpose of prayer [63, 64]. Carefully considered responses that acknowledge and explore the patient's request demonstrate that her concerns have been heard and respect her emotional needs [63, 64]. Understanding and respecting the patients' beliefs in this way may empower them in their support systems and instill confidence in the biopsy team.

During the procedure itself, providing adequate local anesthesia is critical to a successful biopsy and is not optional [54]. As several studies support, pain levels during most imaging-guided breast biopsies are low with use of local anesthesia [23, 26–29]. This might seem obvious when using lower-gauge, large bore needles during core biopsies, but it also holds true for procedures using smaller needles. Satchithananda et al. reported that patients experienced higher levels of pain during fine-needle aspirations (FNA) (using small needles) without local anesthesia, compared to use of much larger needles for ultrasound- and stereotactic-guided core-needle biopsies, where adequate local anesthesia was employed [66]. Likewise, for subdermal lymphoscintigraphy injections, use of local anesthesia resulted in significantly lower pain levels compared to lymphoscintigraphy using no anesthesia [67].

Some patients experience pain during the anesthesia injection itself. When injecting anesthesia into the skin, if the radiologist first touches the sterile area with the gloved finger, indicating the area to be numbed, then patient is less likely to be startled. When raising a skin wheel, a slow injection appears to produce less discomfort than a rapid injection. If she is anxious about the needle stick, having the technologist hold her hand and asking the patient to take slow breaths may focus her mind away from the pain. Buffering lidocaine with sodium bicarbonate (9:1 ratio) has also been shown to reduce the pain of intraparenhcymal anesthesia injections, particularly for women with fatty or scattered fibroglandular tissue, and reduce tissue-sampling pain during ultrasound-guided biopsies [29].

Other interventions can also help to lower biopsy-related anxiety and pain. Bugbee et al. have shown that anxiolytics most effectively reduce anxiety [68]; although anxiolytics or other forms of sedation are not frequently used because recovery space is required, an adult driver is required to accompany the patient, and she would not be to go to work after the procedure. Hypnosis has been shown to alleviate pain during biopsies, although trained personnel are needed to administer the intervention, which would add to the cost [69]. Distraction techniques such as engaging the patient in conversation may be helpful to reduce anxiety, and different studies have shown that listening to music during the procedure can reduce pain and/or anxiety [30, 70]. In addition, studies have shown that mindfulness and loving-kindness-guided meditation practices can significantly reduce anxiety during biopsies [30, 71]. An audio-recorded loving-kindness mediation administered through headphones during the biopsy was shown to also significantly reduce pain levels compared to music and standard care controls and may provide benefit during home use into the peri-surgical period for cancer patients [30, 72].

Conclusion

In conclusion, optimizing patients' experience before, during, and after the breast biopsy is important to the patient-centered approach and involves developing supportive radiologist-patient relationships through enhanced communication, emotional support, and effective interventions. Reducing wait times, providing educational materials or links about biopsy procedures and appointments, and using adequate local anesthesia and other interventions for optimal pain and anxiety control are all important to the patient's biopsy experience. This can lead to greater patient satisfaction and positively influence the patient's own approach to her cancer care journey.

References

1. Mammography Quality Standards Act. https://www.fda.gov/radiation-emittingproducts/mammographyqualitystandardsactandprogram/default.htm. Cited 7 Nov 2018.
2. Breast Imaging Reporting and Data System. https://www.acr.org/Clinical-Resources/Reporting-and-Data-Systems/Bi-Rads. Cited 7 Nov 2018.
3. Aminololama-Shakeri S, Soo MS, Grimm L, et al. Radiologist-patient communication: current practices and barriers to communication in breast imaging. J Am Coll Radiol. 2018; pii: S1546-1440(18)31344–9. https://doi.org/10.1016/j.jacr.2018.10.016. [Epub ahead of print].
4. Seven Dimensions of Patient-Centered Care; Through the Patient's Eyes, Picker Institute, 1993.
5. Jensen JD, et al. Using quality improvement methods to improve patient experience. J Am Coll Radiol. 2016;13:1550–4.
6. Itri JN. Patient-centered radiology. Radiographics. 2015;35:1835–48.
7. Harvey JA, Cohen MA, Brenin DR, Nicholson BT, Adams RB. Breaking bad news: a primer for radiologists in breast imaging. J Am Coll Radiol. 2007;4:800–8.
8. Epstein RM, Street RL. Patient centered communication in cancer care: promoting healing and reducing suffering. National Cancer Institute U.S. Department of Health and Human Services, National Institutes of Health. 2018. https://healthcaredelivery.cancer.gov/pcc/pcc_monograph.pdf. Cited 7 Nov 2018.
9. Ha JF, Anat DS, Longnecker N. Doctor-patient communication: a review. Ochsner J. 2010;10(1):38–43. PMID: 21603354.
10. De Vries AM, de Roten Y, Meystre C, Passchier J, Despland JN, Stiefel F. Clinician characteristics, communication and patient outcome in oncology: a systemic review. Psychooncology. 2014;23(4):275–81.
11. HCAHPS initiative. Available from: https://www.hcahpsonline.org. Cited 1 Sept 2018.
12. Consumer Assessment of Healthcare Providers & Systems (CAHPS). Available from: https://www.cms.gov/Research-Statistics-Data-and-Systems/Research/CAHPS/. Cited 1 Sept 2018.
13. Hobson C. The Economics committee of the patient- and family-centered care commission conducts a survey about patients' imaging expectations, with positive results. 2018. acrbulletin.org/departments/blog/1442-candid-impressions. Cited 7 Nov 2018.

14. Chen MM. It's time for radiology to face the patient. 2018. voiceofradiologyblog. org/2018/08/30/its-time-for-radiology-to-face-the-patient. Cited 7 Nov 2018.
15. Physician Resources for Patient- & Family-Centered Care. Acr.org/Practice-Mangement-Quality-Informatics/Patient-Family-Centered-Care. Cited 24 Oct 2018.
16. Miller LS, Shelby RA, Hayes Balmadrid MA, et al. Patient anxiety before and during imaging-guided breast biopsy procedures: impact of radiologist-patient communication. J Am Coll Radiol. 2013;10:423–31. PMID: 27814826
17. Hayes Balmadrid MA, Shelby RA, Wrenn AA, et al. Anxiety prior to breast biopsy: relationships with length of time from breast biopsy recommendation to biopsy procedure and psychosocial factors. J Health Psychol. 2017;22:561–71. https://doi.org/10.1177/1359105315607828. Epub 2015 Sep 30. PMID: 26424811.
18. Steffens RF, Wright HR, Hester MY, Andrykowski MA. Clinical, demographic, and situational factors linked to distress associated with benign breast biopsy. J Psychosoc Oncol. 2011;29:35–50. https://doi.org/10.1080/07347332.2011.534024. PMID: 21240724.
19. Bailey G. Leading the way in patient interaction: what can breast imagers share with the specialty when it comes to patient communication? ACR Bulletin 2016; https://acrbulletin.org/acr-bulletin-october-2016/761-leading-patient-interaction. Cited 11-7-18.
20. English Oxford Living Dictionaries. https://en.oxforddictionaries.com/definition/anxiety. Cited 7 Nov 2018.
21. Kubler-Ross E. On death and dying: what the dying have to teach doctors, nurses, clergy and their own families. New York: Macmillan; 1969.
22. Trusson D, Pilnick A. The role of hair loss in cancer identity: perceptions of chemotherapy-induced alopecia among women treated for early-stage breast cancer or ductal carcinoma in situ. Cancer Nurs. 2017;40:E9–E16. https://doi.org/10.1097/NCC.0000000000000373.
23. Soo AE, Shelby RS, Miller LS, et al. Predictors of pain during percutaneous imaging-guided core needle biopsies. J Am Coll Radiol. 2014;11:709–16. https://doi.org/10.1016/j.jacr.2014.01.013. PMID: 24993536.
24. Lewin J. Breast imagers can order studies on their patients! SBI Newsl. 2018;3:23–4.
25. Grimm LJ, Shelby RA, Knippa EE, et al. Patient perceptions of breast cancer risk in imaging-detected low-risk scenarios and thresholds for desired intervention: a multi-institution survey. J Am Coll Radiol. 2018;15:911–9. https://doi.org/10.1016/j.jacr.2018.02.010. Epub 2018 Mar 30. PMID: 29606632.
26. Mosier A, Semerad D, Smith D, Rim A, Hammond B. Breast biopsies are minimally painful, exceed patient expectations, and do not represent a genuine lasting harm for most women. Breast J. 2016;22:590–2. https://doi.org/10.1111/tbj.12641. Epub 2016 Jun 27. PMID: 27346578.
27. Pang E, Crystal P, Kulkarni S, Murphy K, Menezes RJ. An audit of pain experienced during image-guided breast biopsy procedures at an Academic Center. Can Assoc Radiol J. 2016;67:250–3. https://doi.org/10.1016/j.carj.2015.10.001. Epub 2016 Jan 30. PMID: 26831731.
28. Seely JM, Hill F, Peddle S, Lau J. An evaluation of patient experience during percutaneous breast biopsy. Eur Radiol. 2017;27:4804–11. https://doi.org/10.1007/s00330-017-4872-2. Epub 2017 May 22. PMID: 28534164.
29. Vasan A, Baker JA, Shelby RA, Soo MSC. Impact of sodium bicarbonate-buffered lidocaine on patient pain during image-guided breast biopsy. J Am Coll Radiol. 2017;14:1194–201. https://doi.org/10.1016/j.jacr.2017.03.026. Epub 2017 May 17. PMID: 28527821.
30. Soo MSC, Jarosz JA, Wren AA, Soo AE, Mowery YM, Johnson KS, Yoon SC, Kim C, Hwang S, Keefe FJ, Shelby RA. Imaging-guided core-needle breast biopsy: impact of meditation and music interventions on patient anxiety, pain and fatigue. J Am Coll Radiol. 2016;13:526–34. PMID: 26853501.
31. Lang EV, Berbaum KS, Lutgendorf SK. Large-core breast biopsy: abnormal salivary cortisol profiles associated with uncertainty of diagnosis. Radiology. 2009;250:631–7. https://doi.org/10.1148/radiol.2503081087. PMID: 19244038.

32. Attai DJ, Hampton R, Staley AC, Borgert A, Landercasper J. What do patients prefer? Understanding patient perspectives on receiving a new breast cancer diagnosis. Ann Surg Oncol. 2016;23:3182–9. https://doi.org/10.1245/s10434-016-5312-2. Epub 2016 Jun 15. PMID: 27306904.

33. Choudhry A, Hong J, Chong K, et al. Patients' preferences for biopsy result notification in an era of electronic messaging methods. JAMA Dermatol. 2015;151:513–21. https://doi.org/10.1001/jamadermatol.2014.5634

34. McElroy JA, Prouix CM, Johnson L, et al. Breaking bad news of a breast cancer diagnosis over the telephone: an emerging trend. Support Care Cancer. 2018; https://doi.org/10.1007/s00520-018-4383-y

35. Portnoy DB. Waiting is the hardest part: anticipating medical test results affects processing and recall of important information. Soc Sci Med. 2010;71:421–8. https://doi.org/10.1016/j.socscimed.2010.04.012. PMID: 20556876.

36. Martinez K, Resnicow K, Williams GC, et al. Does physician communication style impact patient report of decision quality for breast cancer treatment? Patient Educ Couns. 2016;99(12):1947–54.

37. Huysmans Z, Wren AA, Shelby RA, Keefe FJ, Soo MSC. Impact of experiences at the time of breast biopsy on knowledge of recommended follow-up, perceived cancer risk, beliefs about mammography and preferences for support. 35th Annual Meeting & Scientific Sessions of the Society of Behavioral Medicine, Philadelphia, 23–26 April 2014.

38. Kelley JM, Kraft-Todd G, Schapira L, Kossowsky J, Riess H. The influence of the patient-clinician relationship on healthcare outcomes: a systematic review and meta-analysis of randomized controlled trials. PLoS One. 2014;9(4):e94207. PMID: 24718585.

39. Liang W, Burnett CB, Rowland JH, et al. Communication between physicians and older women with localized breast cancer: implications for treatment and patient satisfaction. J Clin Oncol. 2002;20(4):1008–16.

40. Levinson W, Roter DL, Mullooly JP, Dull VT, Frankel RM. Physician-patient communication: the relationship with malpractice claims among primary care physicians and surgeons. JAMA. 1997;277(7):553–9.

41. Beckman HB, Markakis KM, Suchman AL, Frankel RM. The doctor-patient relationship and malpractice: lessons from plaintiff depositions. Arch Intern Med. 1994;154(12):1365–70.

42. Ambady N, LaPlante D, Nguyen T, et al. Surgeons' tone of voice: a clue to malpractice history. Surgery. 2002;132:5–9.

43. Hickson GB, Clayton EW, Githens PB, Sloan FA. Factors that prompted families to file medical malpractice claims following perinatal injuries. JAMA. 1992;267(10):1359–63. https://doi.org/10.1001/jama.1992.03480100065032

44. McWilliam CL, Brown JB, Stewart M. Breast cancer patients' experiences of patient-doctor communication: a working relationship. Patient Educ Cous. 2000;39(2–3):191–204.

45. Henninger, S MSW, LCSW, Ed D, Strategic Services Associate for Duke Primary Care Administration; Duke Medicine; personal communication 2016.

46. Di Blasi Z, Harkness E, Ernst E, Georgiu A, Kleijnen J. Influence of context effects on health outcomes: a systematic review. Lancet. 2001;357:757–62.

47. Wright EB, Hocombe C, Salmon P. Doctors' communication of trust, care, and respect in breast cancer: qualitative study. BMJ. 2004;328:864.

48. Howard. Eleven things patient want from their doctors. Posted 17 February 2017. https://www.practicebuilders.com/blog/11-things-patients-want-from-their-doctors/. Cited 8 Nov 2018.

49. Give the people what they want: 10 things patients say they want from their doctors. NRC Health, 14 April 2016. https://nrchealth.com/10-things-patients-want-from-their-doctors/. Cited 8 Nov 2018.

50. Linver MN. Delivering bad news: a vital skill for professionals involved in breast cancer care. Breast Cancer Online. 2009;12(2):e3.

51. Koropchak CM, Pollak KI, Arnold RM, et al. Studying communication in oncologist-patient encounters: the SCOPE trial. Palliat Med. 2006;20:813–9.

52. Tulsky JA. Interventions to enhance communication among patients, providers, and families. J Palliat Med. 2005;8(Suppl 1):S95–102.
53. RELATE. https://store.healthstream.com/product.aspx?zpid=34388
54. Soo MS, Shelby RA, Johnson KS. Optimizing the patient experience during image-guided breast biopsy. J Breast Imaging. 2019;1(2). https://doi.org/10.1093/jbi/wbz001.
55. Brantley J, Millstine W. Five good minutes. Oakland: New Harbinger Publications; 2005.
56. Cherry K. Understanding body language and facial expressions. Very Well Mind, 16 February 2018. https://www.verywellmind.com/understand-body-language-and-facial-expressions-4147228. Cited 7 Nov 2018.
57. Hale AJ, Freed J, Ricotta D, Farris G, Smith CC. Twelve tips for effective body language for medical educators. Med Teach. 2017;39:914–9.
58. McCorkle R, Ercolano E, Lazenby M, et al. Self-management: enabling and empowering patients living with cancer as a chronic illness. CA Cancer J Clin. 2011;61(1):50–62.
59. Fukui S, Ogawa K, Yamagishi A. Effectiveness of communication skills training of nurses on the quality of life and satisfaction with healthcare professionals among newly diagnosed cancer patients: a preliminary study. Psychooncology. 2011;20(12):1285–91.
60. Rothberg MB, Steele JR, Wheeler J, Arora A, Priya A, Lindenauer PK. The relationship between time spent communicating and communication outcomes on a hospital medicine service. J Gen Intern Med. 2012;27(2):185–9.
61. Hanna MN, Gonzalez-Fernandez M, Barrett AD, Williams KA, Pronovost P. Does patient perception of pain control affect patient satisfaction across surgical units in a tertiary teaching hospital? Am J Med Qual. 2012;27:411–6.
62. Huber DA. Family member presence during procedures. Gastroenterol Nurs. 2006;29(2):174–5.
63. Christensen AR, Cook TE, Arnold RM. How should clinicians respond to requests from patients to participate in prayer? AMA J Ethics. 2018;20(7):E621–9. https://doi.org/10.1001/amajethics.2018.621
64. Kwiatkowski K, Arnold RM, Barnard D. Physicians and prayer requests #120. J Palliat Med. 2011;14(11). https://doi.org/10.1089/jpm.2011.9638
65. McCord G, Cilchrist VJ, Grossman SD, et al. Discussing spirituality with patients: a rational and ethical approach. Ann Fam Med. 2004;2(4):356–61.
66. Satchithananda K, Fernando RA, Ralleigh G, et al. An audit of pain/discomfort experienced during image-guided breast biopsy procedures. Breast J. 2005;11:398–402.
67. Hawkins AS, Yoo DC, Movson JS, Noto RB, Powers K, Baird GL. Administration of subcutaneous buffered lidocaine prior to breast lymphoscintigraphy reduces pain without decreasing lymph node visualization. J Nucl Med Technol. 2014;42:260–4. https://doi.org/10.2967/jnmt.114.144402. Epub 2014 Oct 23.
68. Bugbee ME, Wellisch DK, Arnott IM, et al. Breast core-needle biopsy: clinical trial of relaxation technique versus medication versus no intervention for anxiety reduction. Radiology. 2005;234:73–8. Epub 2004 Nov 24.
69. Lang EV, Berbaum KS, Faintuch S, et al. Adjunctive self-hypnotic relaxation for outpatient medical procedures: a prospective randomized trial with women undergoing large core breast biopsy. Pain. 2006;126:155–64.
70. Téllez A, Sánchez-Jáuregui T, Juárez-García DM, García-SolísInt M. Breast biopsy: the effects of hypnosis and music. Int J Clin Exp Hypn. 2016;64:456–69. https://doi.org/10.1080/00207144.2016
71. Ratcliff CG, Prinsloo S, Chaoul A et al. A randomized controlled trial of brief mindfulness meditation for women undergoing stereotactic breast biopsy. J Am Coll Radiol. 2018; pii: S1546–1440(18)31149–9. https://doi.org/10.1016/j.jacr.2018.09.009. [Epub ahead of print].
72. Wren A, Keefe F, Shelby R et al. Impact of a loving kindness intervention on key outcomes during the perisurgical period of breast cancer. 37th Annual Meeting & Scientific Sessions of the Society of Behavioral Medicine, Washington, DC, 30 March–2 April 2016.

Chapter 2
Ultrasound-Guided Procedures

Amy S. Campbell

Historical Prospective

Image-guided biopsy of mammographically suspicious microcalcifications by means of stereotactic guidance had already been established when the early data reviewing ultrasound-guided, large core percutaneous breast biopsy for sonographically visible lesions was first published in 1993 [1]. The series included 181 lesions, of which 49 went on to surgical excision with 100% agreement. The remaining lesions underwent follow-up with no interval cancers. The average procedure time was 20 minutes and there were no complications. The following year additional studies would evaluate both stereotactic- and ultrasound-guided biopsy, validating the ability of percutaneous biopsy to produce diagnostic results equivalent to that of open surgical biopsy without a surgical scar and decreased time to biopsy and at substantial cost savings [2]. In addition, they touted the ability to provide preoperative counselling to patients, allowing surgeons to plan definitive therapy prior to surgery [3].

Multiple investigators subsequently published studies evaluating the efficacy of ultrasound-guided core needle biopsy. The sensitivity rate was cited between 96% and 98.5% [4–9] with a false-negative rate ranging from 1.6% to 3.9% [5, 7, 9]. Complication rates remained low ranging from 0% to 3% [3, 4, 10–12]. Investigators also made comparisons with open surgical biopsy revealing that ultrasound-guided core needle biopsy could avert surgical excision in 85% of women with benign results with a 56% decrease in the cost of diagnosis [13] and that percutaneous needle biopsy as a means of diagnosis resulted in a single surgical procedure in 84% of women compared to 29% of women undergoing open surgical biopsy [14]. In addition, for women undergoing breast conservation, the likelihood of clear margins after core needle biopsy was 92% compared to only 64% in those women that

A. S. Campbell (✉)
AdventHealth Medical Group - Radiology at Central Florida, Orlando, FL, USA
e-mail: Amy.Campbell.MD@AdventHealth.com

© Springer Nature Switzerland AG 2019
C. M. Kuzmiak (ed.), *Interventional Breast Procedures*,
https://doi.org/10.1007/978-3-030-13402-0_2

underwent open surgical biopsy [15]. The surgical literature published similar supporting data, confirming that patients diagnosed by core needle biopsy were more likely to have negative surgical margins, required fewer surgical procedures for definitive treatment, and allowed for more decisive treatment discussions between patients and their providers prior to surgery [16]. It was the beginning of a diagnostic revolution that would eventually lead percutaneous image-guided biopsy to become the gold standard for the diagnosis of breast cancer.

Fine Needle Aspiration

Fine needle aspiration (FNA) has been a readily available tool to the radiologist for many years. The role of FNA in current breast imaging practices has diminished over time for several reasons. Compared to core needle biopsy, FNA can be plagued by insufficient samples, high false-negative rate, an inability to determine tumor subtype, as well as the need for a qualified breast cytopathologist for proper interpretation [17]. However, this does not mean it no longer has a role in the diagnosis of breast disease. The two most common procedures in which fine needle aspiration is still employed are cyst aspiration and sampling of suspicious lymph nodes not amenable to core biopsy.

Cyst aspiration remains common place for evaluation of cysts lacking benign features and can easily be performed under ultrasound guidance. The goal is to aspirate the cyst to completion to insure adequate sampling (Fig. 2.1). A wide spectrum of cyst fluid can be aspirated, the majority or which can be considered benign and simply discarded. However, fluid that is bloody or blood tinged should always be considered suspicious and submitted for cytologic analysis. It is important to be aware that a small amount of bright red blood can be introduced into the needle hub upon entry into the skin, and this should be differentiated from the cyst fluid itself as it is not a reason for cytologic analysis. In practice it is also advisable that a clip be deployed at the site of any cyst from which suspicious fluid has been aspirated and submitted for cytology. Cysts do not always reaccumulate fluid, and, if excision

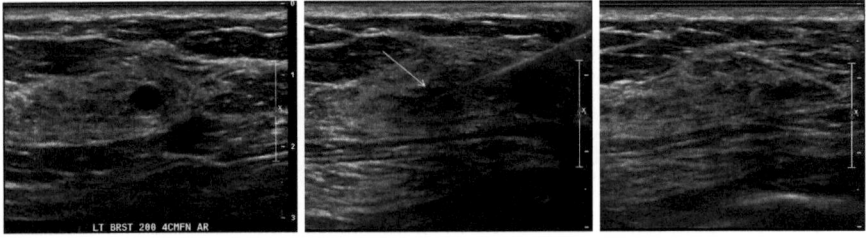

Fig. 2.1 Ultrasound-guided cyst aspiration: cyst prior to aspiration, passage of the needle into the cyst (arrow), and aspiration to completion demonstrated on the post-procedure image

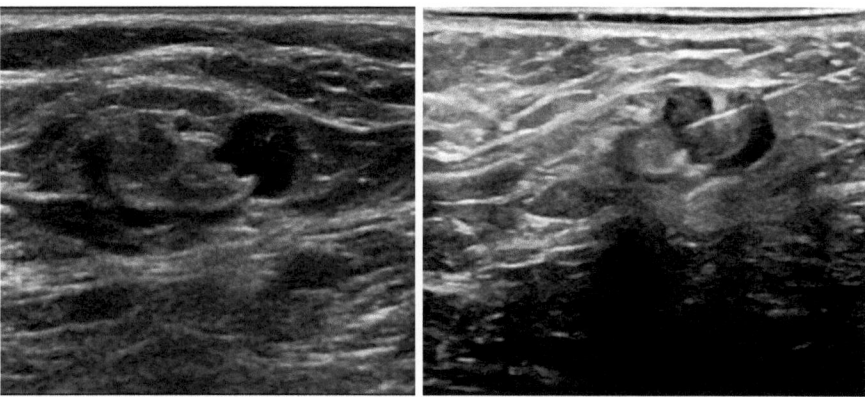

Fig. 2.2 Fine needle aspiration of an abnormal axillary lymph node

is required following the finding of atypical or malignant cells on cytopathology, a tissue marker will be needed for localization at the time of surgery.

Fine needle aspiration also remains a reasonable alternative to core needle biopsy for the sampling of suspicious lymph nodes, particularly when core needle biopsy cannot be performed safely. While cytology lacks the detail of a histologic diagnosis, the added information gained from a positive fine needle aspiration is often sufficient for surgical and oncologic treatment planning. Fine needle aspiration is easily performed utilizing a multi-pass technique with a small gauge needle directed into the lymph node under ultrasound guidance (Fig. 2.2). Ideally fine needle aspiration is performed with real-time, on-site evaluation by a qualified cytopathologist to ensure adequacy of sampling. However, this is not available in many outpatient centers, and knowledge on appropriate handling, preparation, and submission of cytologic aspirates by either the radiologist or support staff is key to ensuring accurate interpretation.

Core Needle Biopsy

Patient Selection

In the words of Dr. Bernard Lown, "Do as much as possible *for* the patient, and as little as possible *to* the patient," this is especially true when performing any interventional procedure. Stereotactic biopsy had already gained wide acceptance when ultrasound-guided procedures were in their infancy, but those that pioneered ultrasound-guided biopsy recognized some key advantages, including lack of ionizing radiation, no need for dedicated equipment, real-time guidance, improved patient comfort, and lower cost [1, 18, 19]. Ultrasound guidance has become the first choice for sampling sonographically visible lesions, even those initially identified mammographically or by MRI, as well as lesions that are clinically palpable [20]. The only contraindications are relative and include close proximity to the chest wall, an underlying breast implant or the inability of a patient to cooperate safely with the procedure.

Preparation

The importance of reviewing both the films and reports prior to performing any biopsy cannot be emphasized enough. The time spent in review ensures proper lesion sampling, prevents errors, and saves time. There are three key components to every pre-procedure assessment: (1) consider what kind of sample you intend to obtain and select the appropriate needle, (2) evaluate your approach, and (3) discuss the plan with your team. In addition, always be mindful of the patient and possible limitations and then make plans to adjust accordingly. Much can be gleaned during the informed consent process, and this time can be invaluable in assuaging patient anxiety and concerns. In addition, limitations related to factors such as patient body habitus can easily be assessed during the pre-procedure ultrasound examination.

Needle Selection

Core needle biopsy can be broken down into three options: semiautomatic, automatic, and vacuum-assisted core needle biopsy. There are multiple vendors offering a variety of needle styles and gauges. The vast majority of clinical trials have reported on utilization of either 14G core needle or 11G vacuum-assisted core needle devices, and both devices remain common place in modern-day breast practices. Device selection is often a matter of personal preference but can also be driven by the nature and location of the lesion to be sampled (Table 2.1).

The semiautomatic core biopsy needle can be a stand-alone device (Fig. 2.3) or a selectable option on a spring-loaded automatic core biopsy needle. Semiautomatic needles are generally offered from 18 to 14G and allow the operator greater control as the needle excursion is deployed in a manual fashion. This level of control makes a popular preference in situations such as sampling of lymph nodes (Fig. 2.4) in

Table 2.1 Needle selection: Comparison of fine needle aspiration, core needle biopsy, and vacuum-assisted core needle biopsy

Needle	FNA	CNB	VACNB
Gauge	25–18G	18–12G	12–7G
Specimen	Cells/fluid	Tissue cores	
Sample technique	Multiple passes		Single pass

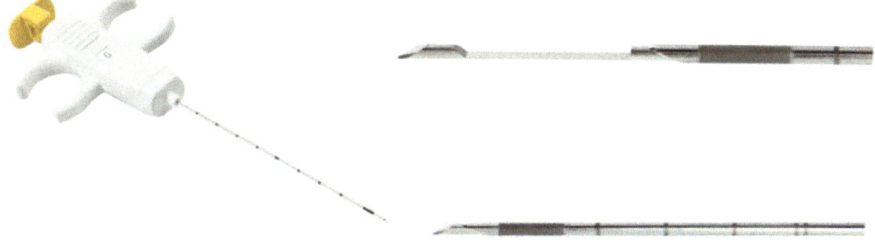

Fig. 2.3 Semiautomatic core needle device

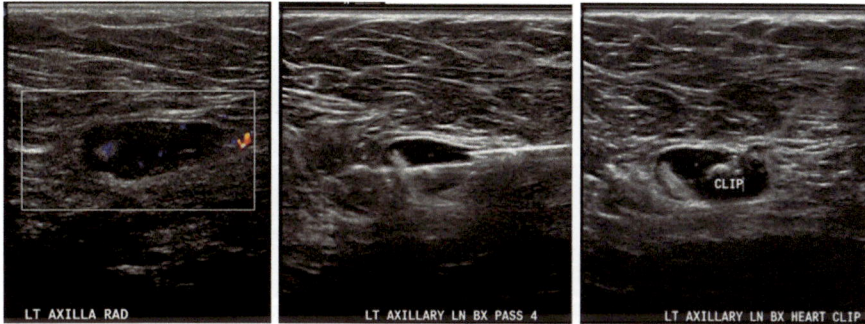

Fig. 2.4 Biopsy of an axillary lymph node with a semiautomatic core biopsy needle demonstrating manual needle excursion with the sample notch in the cortex of the lymph node

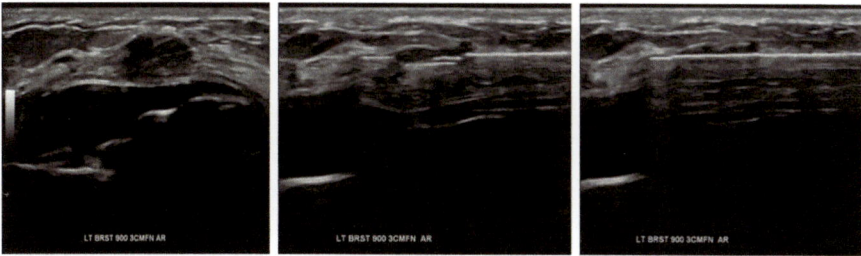

Fig. 2.5 Biopsy of a suspicious mass overlying a breast implant with a semiautomatic core biopsy needle

close proximation to vascular structures or when a lesion closely abuts the surface of a breast implant (Fig. 2.5). The automatic core biopsy needle on the other hand is often considered the workhorse in an active breast practice and generally offered from 16 to 12G with 14G being the most commonly utilized. The automatic core biopsy needle deploys using a spring-loaded device that results in rapid needle excursion which pierces and cuts the lesion in a near simultaneous action (Fig. 2.6).

The popularity of vacuum-assisted core biopsy needles has been driven by the premise of single pass convenience which offers larger cores, reduced likelihood of

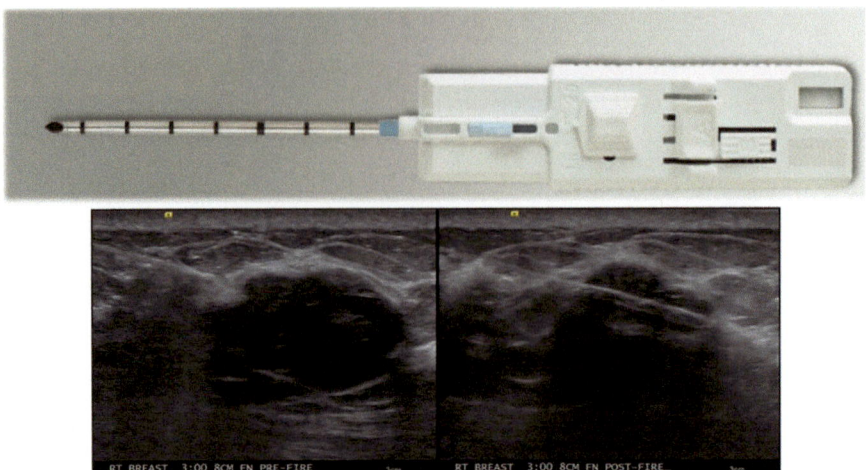

Fig. 2.6 Automatic core biopsy needle which operates via near simultaneous excursion of the sample notch followed by the cutting cannula to obtain a single pass sample

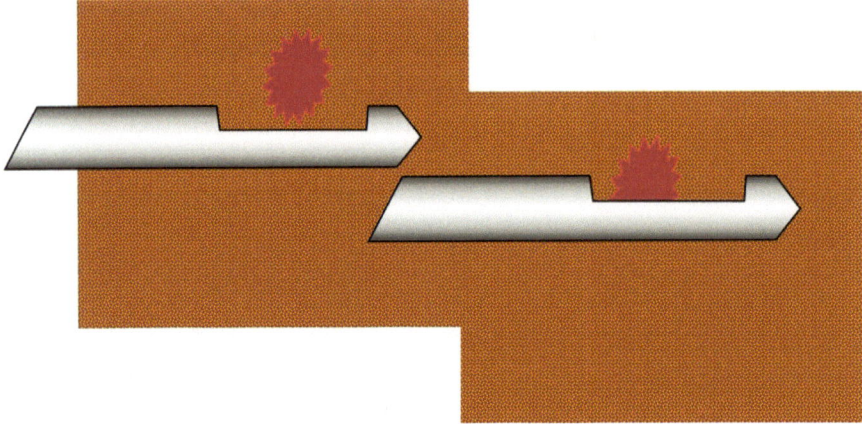

Fig. 2.7 Vacuum-assisted core biopsy needle operates by pulling the lesion into the sample notch while the cutting mechanisms obtains a core, allowing multiple samples to be obtained in a single pass. (Credit: Dag Pavic)

epithelial displacement, and no significant increase in complications [8, 10]. It is important to remember that a direct comparison of 11G vacuum-assisted core needle biopsy and 14G core needle biopsy found that histologic results were similar between the two groups with no significant difference in missed cancers, underestimation of disease, or complications [11]. Vacuum-assisted needles are generally offered from 12 to 7G and allow for single pass, mechanically driven sampling from either one or multiple locations within the same mass (Fig. 2.7).

Technique, Sampling, and Follow-Up

Proper technique for the performance of ultrasound-guided procedures, in particular core needle biopsy, has been detailed extensively in the literature [1, 17, 21] and has become standardized at many facilities. Proper patient positioning is the first and one of the most important steps as it will determine the angle at which the needle is introduced and the distance over which the needle must travel to sample the lesion. Typically, the patient is placed obliquely with the arm over the head to allow the needle to pass parallel to the chest wall. A bolster placed behind that patient's back as well as under the arm is often used to ensure stability and improve patient comfort.

Guidance is typically performed utilizing either a 12–5 MHz or 17–5 MHz linear transducer [22] with selection depending on breast size and lesion depth, and settings such as depth and focal zone should be optimized for lesion visualization with respect to the chest wall. The supply list is similar to other percutaneous biopsy procedures and can be prepared on a case by case basis or customized in a prepared tray (Table 2.2). The tray should be ordered in such a way to allow the radiologist easy access with their free (procedure) hand while maintaining visualization of the lesion with the scanning hand.

Selection of the skin entry site is key to a successful biopsy and will differ according to the depth of the lesion. The fundamental principal being the greater the depth of the lesion the farther the entry point must be from the transducer to allow the needle to maintain parallel orientation with the chest wall over the course of its trajectory (Fig. 2.8). As a general rule of thumb, the entry point for a superficial lesion should be 1–2 cm from the edge of the transducer, while deeper lesions require an entry point slightly farther from the transducer. In the case of a deep lesion, the needle can be advanced at a slightly steeper angle and then lowered into position parallel with the chest wall prior to sampling. The entry point should also permit the needle to remain aligned with the transducer and thus perpendicular to the ultrasound beam to ensure complete visualization during the entire procedure [17, 21] (Fig. 2.9). The needle should also be visualized with respect to surrounding

Table 2.2 Biopsy supply list

Biopsy supply list
Sterile supplies Skin prep Towels Probe cover 4 × 4 gauze
1% lidocaine
Scalpel
Syringe (FNA) or biopsy needle
Marker clip
Specimen container

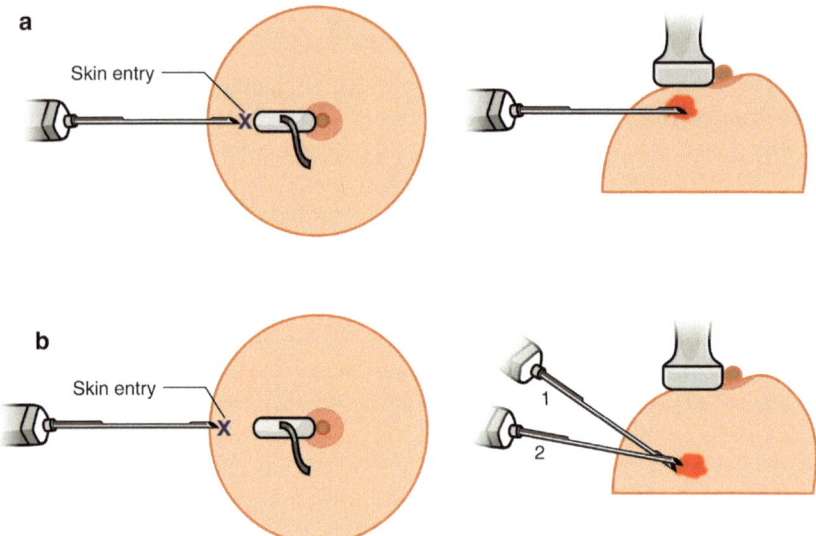

Fig. 2.8 Breast illustration (**a**) Entry point for a superficial mass should be 1–2 cm from the transducer edge. (**b**) Entry point for a deep mass should be farther from the transducer edge (1) to allow the needle to be more easily lowered to parallel once the tip nears the mass (2)

Fig. 2.9 The needle should remain aligned with the ultrasound transducer to allow visualization of the needle tip as it's advanced to the lesion. (Credit: Cherie Kuzmiak)

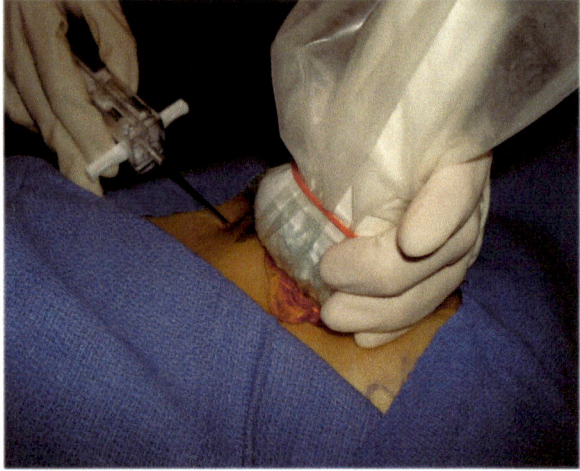

structures prior to sampling to avoid complications such as laceration of a small adjacent artery (Fig. 2.10). Once an entry site is selected, anesthesia is administered at the skin as well as along the biopsy tract to include the tissues surrounding the lesion. This not only allows for administration of adequate anesthetic, but the injection of anesthetic can also be utilized to lift a deep lesion away from the chest wall [17]. In addition, the path of the anesthetic needle permits the operator to visualize and plan the best course of the biopsy needle.

Sampling can be performed with or without an introducer sheath, and the number of times required for needle reentry into the breast depends on the biopsy device that has been selected. A major advantage to the vacuum-assisted device is the need for only a single entry to obtain the necessary samples [10]. The vacuum-assisted needle is typically positioned into or beneath the lesion allowing multiple tissue cores to be pulled down into the sample notch under a single pass (Fig. 2.11). On the other hand, a standard core needle device requires a fresh needle pass to obtain each sample.

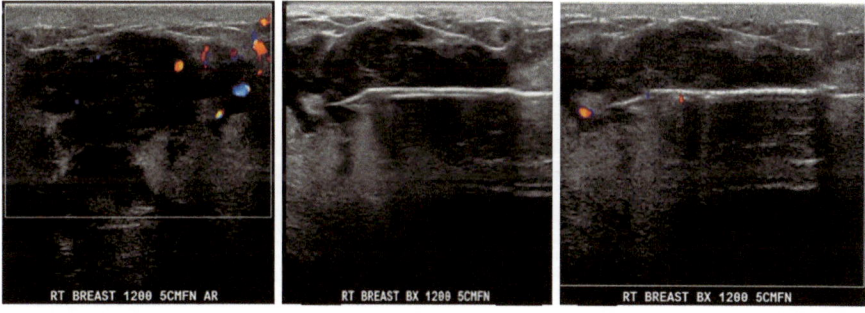

Fig. 2.10 In addition to staying parallel with the chest wall, it is important to visualize the needle at all times and to be aware of adjacent structures such as intertumoral arteries

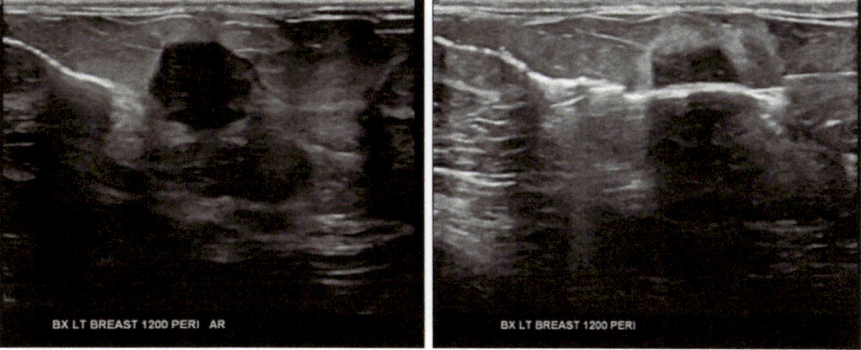

Fig. 2.11 Vacuum-assisted core biopsy needle passed into the mass with the sample notch open prior to sampling, confirming adequate needle position

When using a standard core needle, the use of an introducer sheath can help to maintain easy access to the lesion, particularly in dense-breasted patients or those with deep masses that are difficult to access. However, this is more a matter of radiologist preference than necessity. The standard core needle is typically positioned with the needle tip at the proximal margin of the lesion and the sample notch is then deployed into the mass. Regardless of the method used, it is important to confirm the needle has penetrated the mass to ensure adequate sampling. This can be done by visualizing the needle within the lesion in the selected plane and, if uncertain, confirmed by rotating the probe 90 degrees to obtain an orthogonal image [21].

The number of samples required for adequacy is quite variable in the literature ranging from 3 to 25 cores [5–9, 12, 19, 23]. Clinically, 3–4 core samples are sufficient when utilizing a 14 gauge needle; however, it is important to remember that the quality of the specimens is more important than the actual number obtained. Specifically, samples that are nonfragmented and sink when placed in formalin are more likely to be diagnostic [23]. It is important to always evaluate cores for visual adequacy prior to submission to pathology rather than going simply by the number of samples acquired (Fig. 2.12). Once sampling is complete, a tissue marker should be placed at the biopsy site. Tissue markers serve multiple purposes, including confirmation and correlation with the mammographic finding, marking of the cancer in patients that may require neoadjuvant chemotherapy, and as a way to communicate to other clinicians that a lesion has been sampled.

The final step after every biopsy is radiologic and pathologic concordance. This subject is covered in detail in a later chapter (see Chap. 6). What is important to

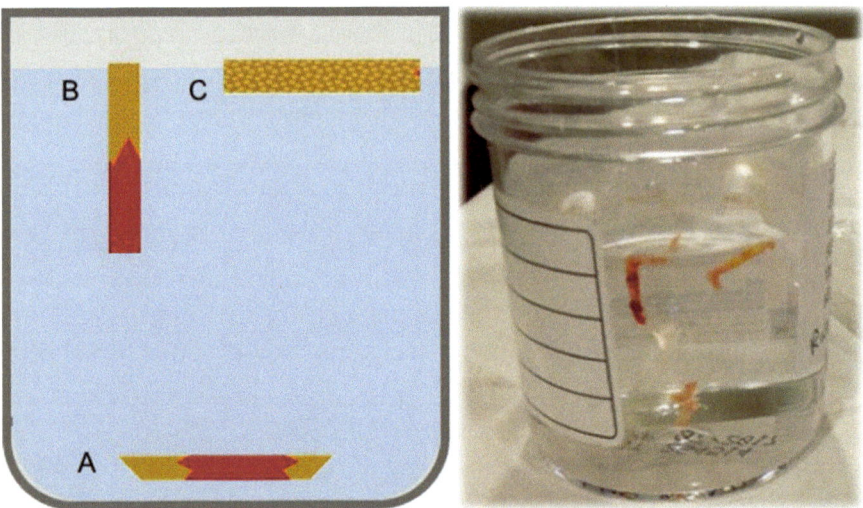

Fig. 2.12 When samples are placed into formalin, they will fall into one of three categories: (**a**) samples that sink because they are comprised mostly of tissue from the lesion in question; (**b**) samples that partially sink, a mixture of the lesion and surrounding fat; and (**c**) samples that float, fat with little to no tissue from the lesion. (Credit: Dag Pavic)

remember, is that the cornerstone to every successful biopsy practice is a radiologist that understands the significance of accurate concordance reporting. The radiologist plays an integral role in the appropriate care and follow-up of all biopsy patients.

Needle and Radioactive Seed Localization

Needle Localization

Patients diagnosed with high-risk lesions or malignancy amenable to breast conserving therapy will ultimately undergo surgical excision. Lesions that were sampled under ultrasound guidance are often able to undergo preoperative localization with ultrasound unless the lesion was obliterated during initial sampling or the patient has undergone neoadjuvant chemotherapy. This is particularly beneficial in the fasting patient that can be more prone to vasovagal reaction during localization under mammography which requires the patient to be upright and under compression. As with core biopsy needles, there are a variety of wire localization systems available, and selection is a matter of radiologist or in some cases surgeon preference. The goal of wire localization is to guide the surgeon to the lesion over the shortest distance possible to produce the best overall cosmetic outcome for the patient. Most radiologists find this much easier to achieve under ultrasound guidance as there is more flexibility in the selection of needle approach.

Preparations and approach to preoperative lesion localization under ultrasound guidance are nearly the same as those for biopsy. In ultrasound-guided needle/wire localization, the needle should be advanced through the lesion under ultrasound guidance. To ensure accurate positioning of the wire following deployment, the tip of the needle should pass 5–10 mm beyond the distal aspect of the lesion. This allows placement of the hook beyond the lesion with the thick or beaded portion of the wire within the lesion following wire deployment (Fig. 2.13).

Radioactive Seed Localization

Placement of a radioactive seed is similar in principle to placement of a localization wire, with an Iodine 125 seed deployed through a needle system (Fig. 2.14). The needle is guided into the central portion of the lesion where the radioactive seed can be deployed under direct visualization to ensure accurate placement. The salient difference in the placement of a radioactive seed is also one of its major benefits; the approach with respect to distance from the lesion is much less important, and with the absence of an external wire, the radioactive seed allows the surgeon to make their incision at the location of their choice without concerns about wire retrieval [24].

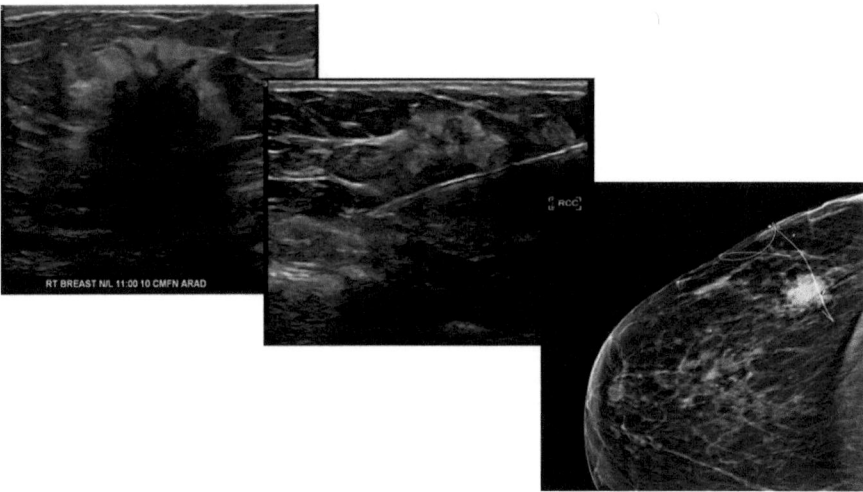

Fig. 2.13 Ultrasound-guided needle localization

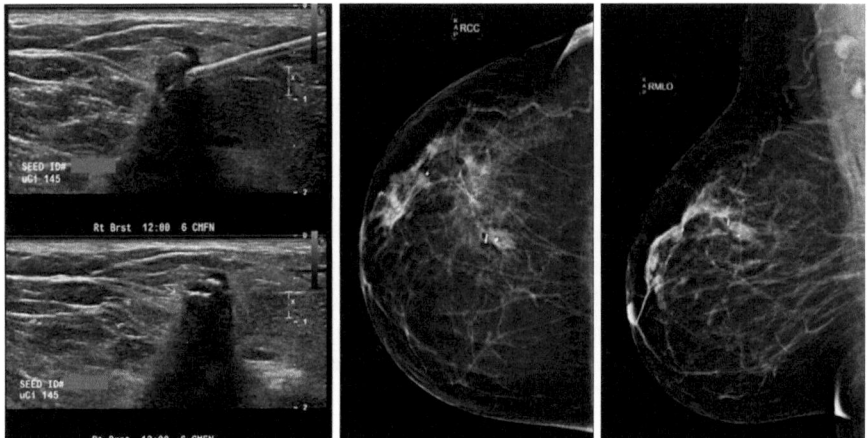

Fig. 2.14 Ultrasound-guided radioactive seed localization

References

1. Parker SH, Jobe WE, Dennis MA, Stavros AT, Johnson KK, Yakes WF, et al. US-guided auto-mated large-core breast biopsy. Radiology. 1993;187(2):507–11.
2. Parker SH. Percutaneous large core breast biopsy. Cancer. 1994;74(1 Suppl):256–62.
3. Parker SH, Burbank F, Jackman RJ, Aucreman CJ, Cardenosa G, Cink TM, et al. Percutaneous large-core breast biopsy: a multi-institutional study. Radiology. 1994;193(2):359–64.
4. Bruening W, Fontanarosa J, Tipton K, Treadwell JR, Launders J, Schoelles K. Systematic review: comparative effectiveness of core-needle and open surgical biopsy to diagnose breast lesions. Ann Intern Med. 2010;152(4):238–46.

5. Sauer G, Deissler H, Strunz K, Helms G, Remmel E, Koretz K, et al. Ultrasound-guided large-core needle biopsies of breast lesions: analysis of 962 cases to determine the number of samples for reliable tumour classification. Br J Cancer. 2005;92(2):231–5.
6. Schoonjans JM, Brem RF. Fourteen-gauge ultrasonographically guided large-core needle biopsy of breast masses. J Ultrasound Med. 2001;20(9):967–72.
7. Schueller G, Jaromi S, Ponhold L, Fuchsjaeger M, Memarsadeghi M, Rudas M, et al. US-guided 14-gauge core-needle breast biopsy: results of a validation study in 1352 cases. Radiology. 2008;248(2):406–13.
8. Simon JR, Kalbhen CL, Cooper RA, Flisak ME. Accuracy and complication rates of US-guided vacuum-assisted core breast biopsy: initial results. Radiology. 2000;215(3):694–7.
9. Youk JH, Kim EK, Kim MJ, Oh KK. Sonographically guided 14-gauge core needle biopsy of breast masses: a review of 2,420 cases with long-term follow-up. AJR Am J Roentgenol. 2008;190(1):202–7.
10. Parker SH, Klaus AJ, McWey PJ, Schilling KJ, Cupples TE, Duchesne N, et al. Sonographically guided directional vacuum-assisted breast biopsy using a handheld device. AJR Am J Roentgenol. 2001;177(2):405–8.
11. Philpotts LE, Hooley RJ, Lee CH. Comparison of automated versus vacuum-assisted biopsy methods for sonographically guided core biopsy of the breast. AJR Am J Roentgenol. 2003;180(2):347–51.
12. Smith DN, Rosenfield Darling ML, Meyer JE, Denison CM, Rose DI, Lester S, et al. The utility of ultrasonographically guided large-core needle biopsy: results from 500 consecutive breast biopsies. J Ultrasound Med. 2001;20(1):43–9.
13. Liberman L, Feng TL, Dershaw DD, Morris EA, Abramson AF. US-guided core breast biopsy: use and cost-effectiveness. Radiology. 1998;208(3):717–23.
14. Liberman L, LaTrenta LR, Dershaw DD, Abramson AF, Morris EA, Cohen MA, et al. Impact of core biopsy on the surgical management of impalpable breast cancer. AJR Am J Roentgenol. 1997;168(2):495–9.
15. Liberman L, LaTrenta LR, Dershaw DD. Impact of core biopsy on the surgical management of impalpable breast cancer: another look at margins. AJR Am J Roentgenol. 1997;169(5):1464–5.
16. White RR, Halperin TJ, Olson JA Jr, Soo MS, Bentley RC, Seigler HF. Impact of core-needle breast biopsy on the surgical management of mammographic abnormalities. Ann Surg. 2001;233(6):769–77.
17. Parker SH, Burbank F. A practical approach to minimally invasive breast biopsy. Radiology. 1996;200(1):11–20.
18. Liberman L. Centennial dissertation. Percutaneous imaging-guided core breast biopsy: state of the art at the millennium. AJR Am J Roentgenol. 2000;174(5):1191–9.
19. Margolin FR, Leung JW, Jacobs RP, Denny SR. Percutaneous imaging-guided core breast biopsy: 5 years' experience in a community hospital. AJR Am J Roentgenol. 2001;177(3):559–64.
20. Liberman L, Ernberg LA, Heerdt A, Zakowski MF, Morris EA, LaTrenta LR, et al. Palpable breast masses: is there a role for percutaneous imaging-guided core biopsy? AJR Am J Roentgenol. 2000;175(3):779–87.
21. Youk JH, Kim EK, Kim MJ, Lee JY, Oh KK. Missed breast cancers at US-guided core needle biopsy: how to reduce them. Radiographics. 2007;27(1):79–94.
22. Hooley RJ, Scoutt LM, Philpotts LE. Breast ultrasonography: state of the art. Radiology. 2013;268(3):642–59.
23. Fishman JE, Milikowski C, Ramsinghani R, Velasquez MV, Aviram G. US-guided core-needle biopsy of the breast: how many specimens are necessary? Radiology. 2003;226(3):779–82.
24. Goudreau SH, Joseph JP, Seiler SJ. Preoperative radioactive seed localization for nonpalpable breast lesions: technique, pitfalls, and solutions. Radiographics. 2015;35(5):1319–34.

Chapter 3
DBT-Guided Biopsy

Stamatia Destounis, Andrea Arieno, and Amanda Santacroce

Introduction

Core needle biopsy has been utilized routinely in clinical practice for years as the method of choice to sample suspicious lesions detected on breast imaging. The procedure has been proven to be a safe, accurate, and less invasive alternative to surgical excision, as well as more cost-effective for the patient. Digital breast tomosynthesis (DBT) was introduced to the mammography market in 2011, when the first DBT device received Food and Drug Administration (FDA) approval. Since that time, the technology has been the subject of much investigative research, evaluating its use in both screening and diagnostic settings. Multiple studies have reported decreased recall rates and increased breast cancer detection rates of 1.2–2.7 per 1000 [1–7]; increases have been found in invasive cancer detection (40–41%) without significant increase in ductal carcinoma in situ (DCIS) detection [2, 4].

DBT use in clinical practice continues to grow; nationally as of October 2018, there are more than 4700 certified facilities with DBT units and more than 6600 accredited DBT units [8]. DBT is being utilized in all practice types and in a variety of exam and patient indications [9]. With this growth comes scenarios in which a suspicious lesion is identified only on DBT imaging, without an ultrasound (US) correlate, creating a management dilemma for the radiologist; these scenarios can be addressed by use of tomosynthesis-guided core biopsy.

S. Destounis (✉) · A. Arieno · A. Santacroce
Elizabeth Wende Breast Care, LLC, Rochester, NY, USA
e-mail: sdestounis@ewbc.com

© Springer Nature Switzerland AG 2019
C. M. Kuzmiak (ed.), *Interventional Breast Procedures*,
https://doi.org/10.1007/978-3-030-13402-0_3

Practical Considerations Prior to Implementation

Prior to implementation, a facility must do thorough investigation. There are details which need to be considered for the incorporation of DBT-guided biopsy into the clinical workflow to go smoothly. There are two options clinically available for DBT-guided core needle biopsy: DBT biopsy prone or upright DBT biopsy. When making the decision for which system is right for a practice, financials, patient volume, and space considerations are all key factors.

A facility should determine if it will incorporate DBT biopsy from the start of using DBT imaging or if it will delay DBT biopsy integration until DBT mammography volume increases.

The number of DBT units in the practice is also an important consideration. The upright system is often selected due to the simplicity of implementation in comparison to the prone table, as the upright biopsy system can be added onto an already existing DBT system, thus not requiring a dedicated space, unlike the prone table. In addition, the upright system is less of a financial investment than a prone table, making the upright option a more feasible choice for smaller practices. An important drawback to consider is that the mammography room will now need to be available for interventional procedures aside from just mammography imaging, which can cause interruption in the clinic workflow.

If a facility already utilizes DBT for mammography imaging, has a large volume, and/or has a stereotactic biopsy table already in use, transition to prone DBT biopsy may be a better option. The learning curve for technologists and physicians will likely be small. The software and user interface have a similar appearance to DBT mammography units, making the transition easier. For larger practices with high patient volume, it is likely worth the additional cost and space to invest in a dedicated prone table to avoid interruption to screening workflow.

The DBT-Guided Biopsy Procedure

In general, the DBT-guided procedure is like stereotactic biopsy. The approach is planned as would be done traditionally, based on the location of the lesion. The procedure that follows is based on performing a DBT-guided biopsy utilizing the prone table.

The patient is positioned prone on the biopsy table, and the lesion is (ideally) centered in the biopsy window with the shortest skin to lesion distance, to allow the biopsy needle to travel through the least amount of breast tissue (Fig. 3.1a–b). A tomosynthesis scout image is acquired, and on the screen, the user scrolls through the images to identify the appropriate image slice of the lesion to be biopsied. X, Y, and Z values will automatically appear once lesion is clicked; this will create the target for the procedure to move forward (Fig. 3.2a–b). This process

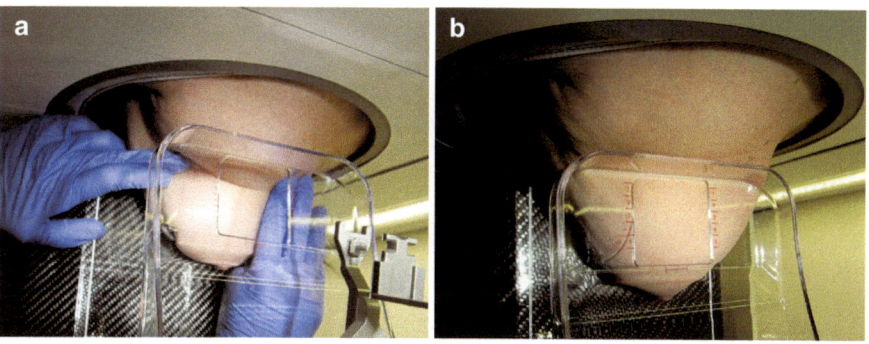

Fig. 3.1 (**a–b**) Positioning the breast for lesion targeting at the start of the biopsy procedure

replaces the traditional targeting for stereotactic biopsy, which requires the scout and stereo pair images to identify the Z. In a situation with multiple lesions, you can repeat this process for multiple targets (up to 12) using the *Multi-pass* button. The technologist performing the procedure can see the coordinates selected before proceeding with the procedure (Fig. 3.3a–b). Once the biopsy needle is in place, the tomosynthesis pre-fire image is acquired. Some facilities may acquire 2D stereo pre-fire images. At this time, it is important for the user to scroll through to verify that the needle is positioned accurately at the lesion of interest; this also allows for time to make any necessary needle adjustments. Sampling of the lesion then occurs as is done traditionally, as well as for the clip placement, and specimen imaging (if applicable). A post-fire tomosynthesis image is then obtained; again, the user can scroll through the projection images to identify the lesion and ensure accurate sampling.

Management of DBT Findings with DBT VAB

When does DBT-guided biopsy help? This can be situational; is the lesion seen by DBT only? Is there an ultrasound correlate? Ultrasound is the first line of imaging after mammography for a DBT-only finding. When an US correlate is present, an US-guided core needle biopsy can be performed for tissue diagnosis. However, when there is no US correlate, additional options must be investigated. It is preferable to perform biopsy by the modality that best demonstrates the lesion, making the availability of DBT-guided biopsy crucial. With the increased use of DBT in the screening setting, radiologists will more frequently encounter situations of asymptomatic women with 2D mammographically occult lesions. Studies have shown that these lesions visible on DBT-only are likely to be atypical or malignant, making it essential to have a way to histologically sample these lesions [10–11]. Prior to the availability of DBT-guided biopsy, management of findings with no US correlate

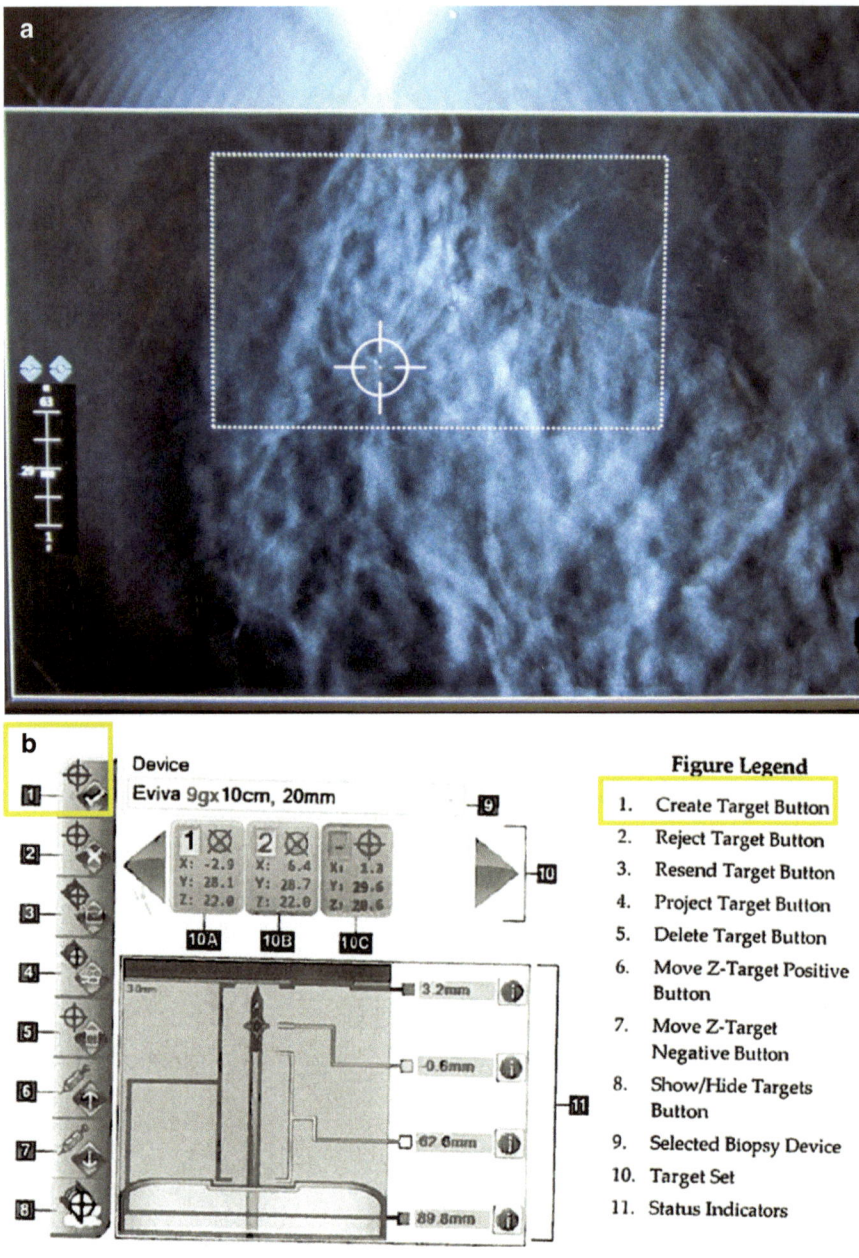

Fig. 3.2 (a–b) Identifying and creating the target to sample the lesion of interest

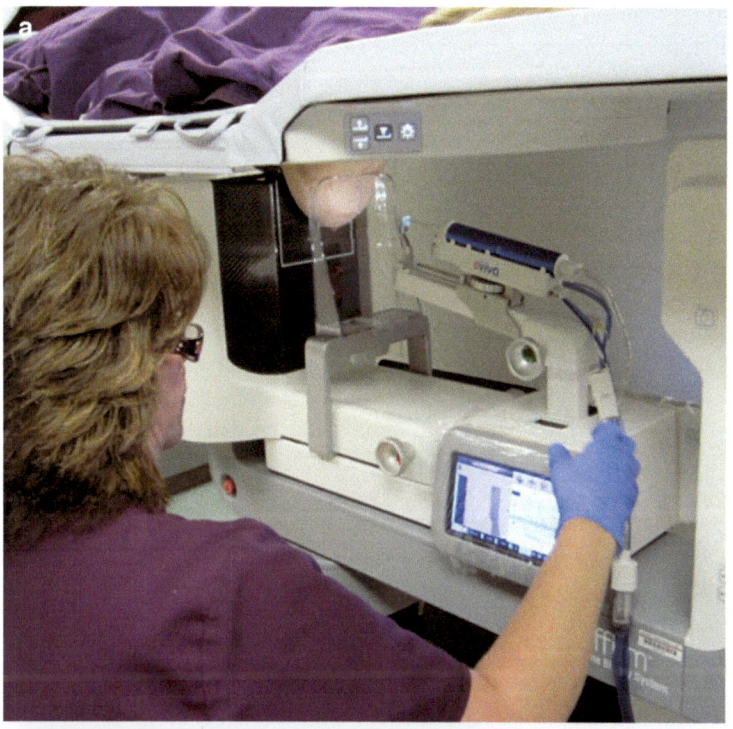

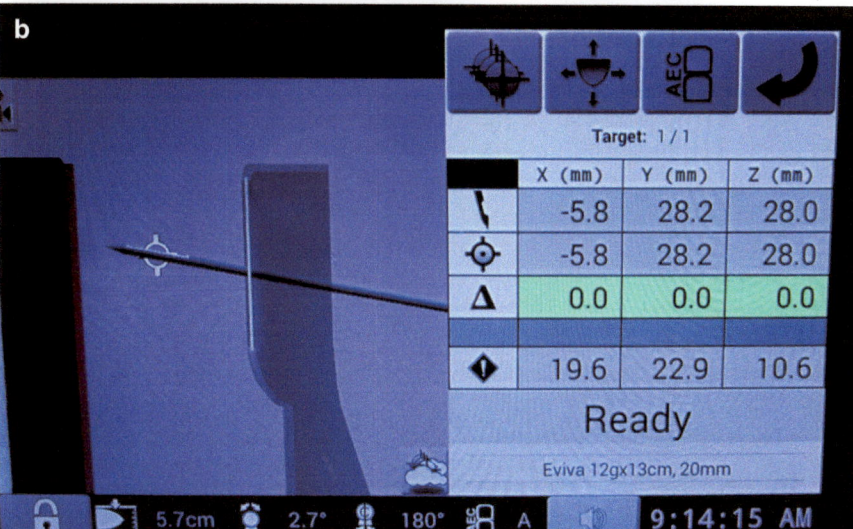

Fig. 3.3 (a–b) Sending X, Y, Z coordinates to the biopsy console to initiate the biopsy procedure

was problematic. Frequently, DBT-guided wire localization was performed before surgical excision; this method was proven to be an accurate and feasible alternative to sample DBT-only lesions [12].

DBT-guided biopsy research has progressed from wire localization to vacuum-assisted biopsy, and several investigations have proven it is a practicable and reliable method to sample breast lesions. Studies have found that DBT VAB can offer better lesion localization by 3D nature of the technology of both low-contrast masses and distortions [12, 13]. Waldherr et al. evaluated the feasibility and performance of (upright) DBT-guided VAB compared to stereo (SVAB) and found that all TVAB biopsies were technically successful and obtained the targeted lesion (microcalcifications) in 100% of cases; SVAB did not obtain the targeted microcalcifications in 1/86 [14]. Distortions were exclusively biopsied with TVAB resulting in 13 malignant diagnoses and 11 radial scars/complex sclerosing lesions. The mean size of the distortions was less than 1 cm, demonstrating that TVAB can sample small lesions with accuracy. DBT VAB had superior performance in comparison with PS VAB in a clinical evaluation by Schrading et al.; DBT VAB had a 100% technical success rate, versus 93% for PS VAB [13]. Reidentifying and targeting lesions during PS VAB took longer than it did during DBT VAB (P, 0.0001), and time for tissue sampling was about the same for both methods ($P = 0.067$). These findings give the clinician the confidence needed to pursue the adoption of DBT-guided biopsy.

Detection of architectural distortion (AD) has increased with use of DBT imaging and is increasingly a finding visualized only on DBT (Fig. 3.4a–d). While there is limited data reported on in the literature on the outcomes of these distortions that are detected on DBT and occult on FFDM and US, several authors have described their individual experience (Table 3.1). Patel et al. reported the experience of DBT VAB of AD that was occult at 2D mammography and ultrasound, finding DBT VAB to be a reliable, minimally invasive method with the ability to detect carcinoma [15]. DBT-guided biopsy was successful in 100% of cases, with 26% PPV (9/34). Sixteen radial scars were diagnosed, nearly half of the benign lesions. Bahl et al. reported similar findings; radial scar was the most common benign pathologic finding associated with AD at both 2D mammography and DBT but was significantly more common at DBT [16] (Fig. 3.5a–c). The study found that the presence of distortion on mammography and no US correlate was less likely to represent malignancy than AD with an US correlate. The proportion of high-risk lesions that upgrade to invasive disease is higher with DBT than with digital mammography [18]; with the increase in detection of some of these high-risk lesions (i.e., radial scars), this demonstrates the importance of being able to adequately sample lesions detected on DBT.

Pearls and Pitfalls of DBT-Guided Biopsy

As with any procedure, there are benefits and challenges to implementation and use. DBT-guided biopsy is no exception.

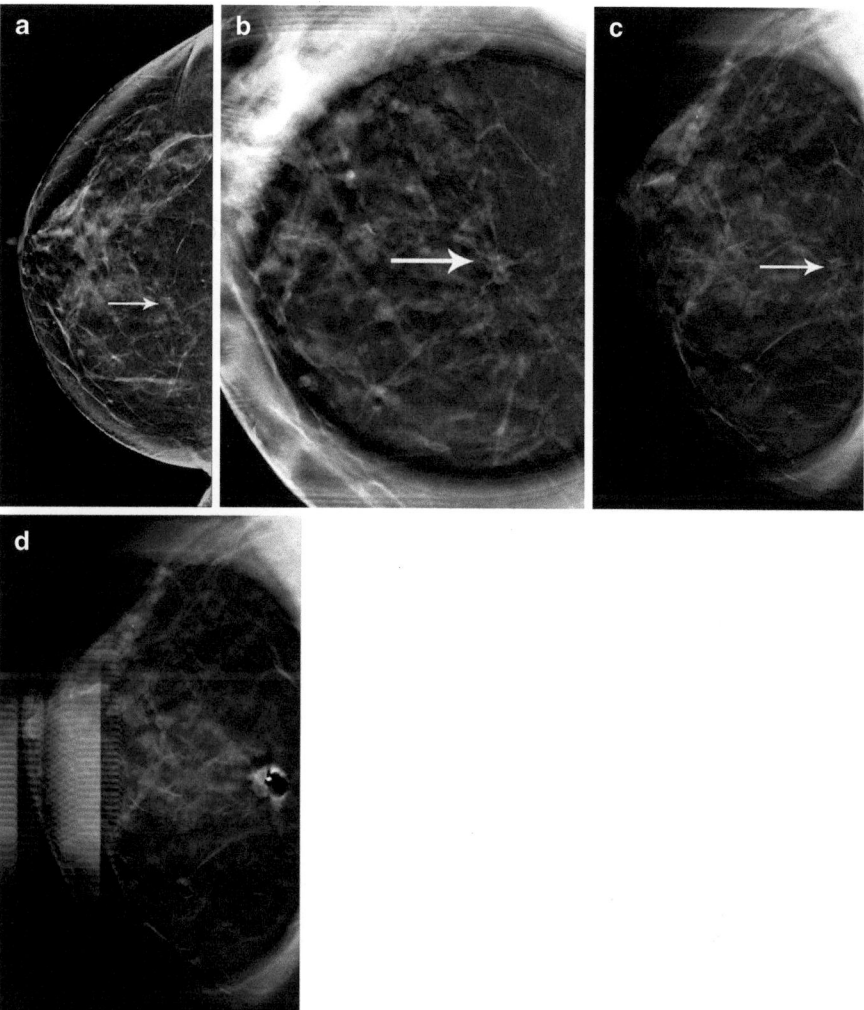

Fig. 3.4 (**a–d**) 53-year-old patient presented for screening mammography. Architectural distortion was seen on the RCC view (**a**, arrow), best demonstrated on the DBT slices as demonstrated on the spot view (**b**, arrow). DBT-guided biopsy was recommended, and the area was targeted on the pre-biopsy scouting image (**c**, arrow), resulting in a successful biopsy procedure (**d**). Pathology results revealed a diagnosis of grade 1 Invasive ductal carcinoma

Table 3.1 Reported PPVs of DBT-detected lesions biopsied under DBT-guided biopsy guidance

	Number of DBT biopsied lesions	Types of lesions	PPV
Patel et al. [15]	34	AD	26%
Waldherr et al. [14]	148	AD, Calcs	30%
Ray et al. [10]	14	AD	35.7%
Freer et al. [12]	36	AD	47.2%
Bahl et al. [16]	274	AD	50.7%
Partyka et al. [17]	19	AD	44.4%

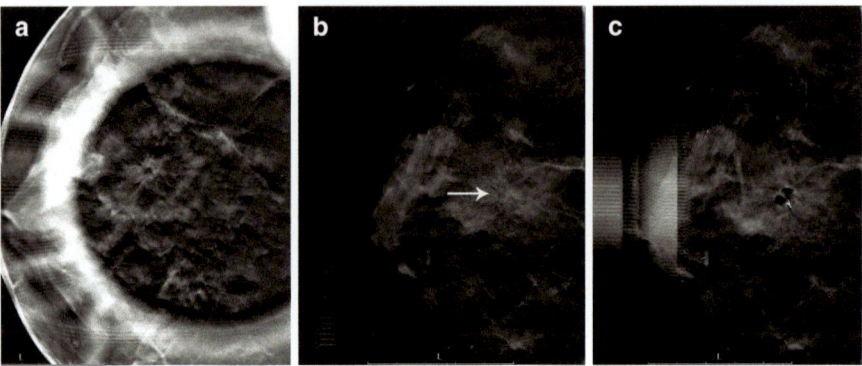

Fig. 3.5 (**a–c**) 55-year-old patient presented for screening mammography. Architectural distortion was noted in the right superior breast (**a**), best identified on the DBT slices. DBT-guided biopsy was recommended, and the lesion of interested was targeted and sampled successfully (arrow, **b–c**), with pathology revealing a diagnosis of radial scar. Surgical excision was recommended; pathology at excision was radial scar

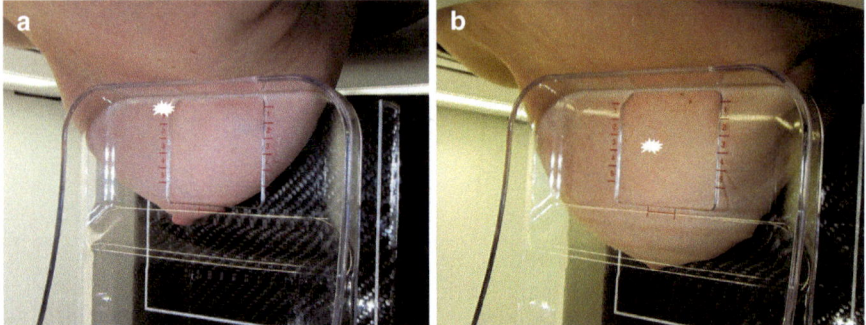

Fig. 3.6 (**a–b**) The clear compression paddle used for the biopsy procedure allows for easier re-scouting of the targeted lesion

Advantages

The primary benefit of DBT-guided biopsy is the ability to biopsy lesions visualized only on DBT imaging, allowing for immediate tissue sampling and diagnosis verses referring the patient for surgical biopsy. Additionally, the DBT biopsy systems come with a clear compression paddle, allowing for faster re-scouting (Fig. 3.6a–b).

The upright DBT system may be more comfortable for patients; it has been reported that there is improved comfort for patients with back pain, respiratory problems, or difficult with prone positioning [19]. The upright system can also allow for greater access to sampling far posterior lesions. Additionally, as mentioned previously, this option can be added to existing DBT equipment, which saves space and is less of a capital expense.

Prone DBT biopsy advantages include the ability to access posterior tissue – the table comes with a top panel that can be removed to allow for greater access to posterior lesions. The panel can also be removed to accommodate patient body habitus and allow for greater patient comfort. There is reduced chance of a vasovagal reaction with prone biopsy and, in addition, elimination of any impact on the imaging workflow with mammography rooms due to the table being in a designated intervention room.

Due to the improved lesion visualization with DBT, there are advantages with lesion visibility, visualizing vasculature, and vessel identification. Mesurolle has described the benefit with the ability to avoid large vessels, which ultimately can avoid causing a hematoma [20]. The nature of the DBT technology allows for improved targeting, with more accurate localization within the 3D volume, leading to improved biopsy performance with reduction in complication rate.

Several studies have reported faster biopsy times with DBT-guided biopsy in comparison to traditional stereotactic biopsy (Table 3.2). This is a benefit for the patient, as decreased procedure time will contribute to a better experience for the patient. Patient movement during the procedure can be minimized, reducing the potential need for repeat imaging/biopsy. Contributing to the decreased procedure time is the fact that there are fewer exposures needed to complete the procedure; for example, you do not need to take stereo pair images. Smith et al. reported that there was a less number of attempts needed to position with DBT, and in total, upright DBT consisted of 7.45 images, prone stereotactic, 10.08 ($P < 0.0001$) [21].

Disadvantages

The DBT biopsy procedure comes with similar disadvantages to any stereotactic biopsy, including bleeding, lidocaine obscuring the lesion. In such situations, it is important to trust your targeting prior to bleeding or lidocaine.

Biopsy of posterior lesions can be difficult when utilizing the prone table, a disadvantage of this approach in comparison to utilizing the upright biopsy system.

The upright approach comes with its own challenges, including the chance of patients experiencing a vasovagal reaction due to the upright positioning and chance of the patient seeing the needle/biopsy procedure. Additionally, with use of the upright biopsy system, there are operational considerations. Utilizing a mammography unit for biopsy limits use of the machine for screening or imaging diagnostic patients. This can be addressed by scheduling biopsies in batches or creating specific biopsy slots in a schedule.

Table 3.2 Comparison of procedure times

	Avg. procedure time DBT VAB	Avg. procedure time PS VAB
Schrading et al. [13]	13 minutes	29 minutes
Waldherr et al. [14]	15.4 minutes	23 minutes
Smith et al. [21]	27 minutes	30 minutes

Tips and Tricks

Performing DBT-guided biopsy is, for the most part, a similar procedure to performing stereotactic guided biopsy; thus, the experienced core biopsy technologist will have a small learning curve. Regardless, with more experience performing DBT-guided biopsies, several situations may arise that allow for staff learning a specific tip or trick to assist others. For example, after targeting the lesion, and administering lidocaine, the field of view can become obscured, leading to biopsy staff questioning if the lesion of interest is still in view. It is important to trust your initial targeting and do not attempt to retarget at this point. Additionally, when a scout image is obtained and the area of interest is not seen in the biopsy window but can be seen through the clear paddle, the depth can still be checked to determine if the approach chosen will be suitable or if a different direction will be needed for accurate tissue sampling to occur.

Conclusions

As the use of DBT becomes more widespread, it will be beneficial for radiologists to become more comfortable and familiar with DBT-guided biopsies. The technique has shown to be a safe, effective, and reliable method for tissue sampling and is an important element to incorporate in a breast imaging practice offering DBT imaging.

References

1. Rafferty EA, Park JM, Philpotts LE, Poplack SP, Sumkin JH, Halpern EF, Niklason LT. Assessing radiologist performance using combined digital mammography and breast tomosynthesis compared with digital mammography alone: results of a multicenter, multireader trial. Radiology. 2013;266(1):104–13.
2. Skaane P, Bandos AI, Gullien R, et al. Comparison of digital mammography alone and digital mammography plus tomosynthesis in a population-based screening program. Radiology. 2013;267:47–56.
3. Ciatto S, Houssami N, Bernardi D, et al. Integration of 3D digital mammography with tomosynthesis for population breast-cancer screening (STORM): a prospective comparison study. Lancet Oncol. 2013;14:583–9.
4. Friedewald SM, Rafferty EA, Rose SL, et al. Breast cancer screening using tomosynthesis in combination with digital mammography. JAMA. 2014;311:2499–507.
5. Rose SL, Tidwell AL, Bujnoch LJ, Kushwaha AC, Nordmann AS, Sextron R Jr. Implementation of breast tomosynthesis in a routine screening practice: an observational study. AJR. 2013;200:1401–8.
6. Durand MA, Haas BM, Yao X, et al. Early clinical experience with digital breast tomosynthesis for screening mammography. Radiology. 2015;274:85–92.

7. Sharpe RE, Venkataraman S, Phillips J, et al. Increased cancer detection rate and variations in the recall rate resulting from implementation of 3D digital breast tomosynthesis into a population-based screening program. Radiology. 2016;278:698–706.
8. MQSA National Statistics. Accessed at https://www.fda.gov/Radiation-EmittingProducts/MammographyQualityStandardsActandProgram/FacilityScorecard/ucm113858.htm
9. Gao Y, Babb JS, Toth HK, Moy L, Heller SL. Digital breast tomosynthesis practice patterns following 2011 FDA approval: a survey of breast imaging radiologists. Acad Radiol. 2017;24(8):947–53.
10. Ray KM, Turner E, Sickles EA, Joe BN. Suspicious findings at digital breast tomosynthesis occult to conventional digital mammography: imaging features and pathology findings. Breast J. 2015;21(5):538–42.
11. Viala J, Gignier P, Perret B, et al. Stereotactic vacuum-assisted biopsies on a digital breast 3D-tomosynthesis system. Breast J. 2012;19(1):4–9.
12. Freer PE, Niell B, Rafferty EA. Preoperative tomosynthesis-guided needle localization of mammographically and sonographically occult breast lesions. Radiology. 2015;275:377–83.
13. Schrading S, Distelmaier M, Dirrichs T, et al. Digital breast tomosynthesis-guided vacuum-assisted breast biopsy: initial experiences and comparison with prone stereotactic vacuum-assisted biopsy. Radiology. 2015;274(3):654–62.
14. Waldherr C, Berclaz G, Altermatt HJ, et al. Tomosynthesis-guided vacuum-assisted breast biopsy: a feasibility study. Eur Radiol. 2016;26:1582–9.
15. Patel BK, Covington M, Pizzitola VJ, et al. Initial experience of tomosynthesis-guided vacuum-assisted biopsies of tomosynthesis-detected (2D mammography and ultrasound occult) architectural distortion. AJR. 2018;210:1–6.
16. Bahl M, Lamb LR, Lehman CD. Pathologic outcomes of architectural distortion on digital 2D versus tomosynthesis mammography. AJR. 2017;209:1162–7.
17. Partyka L, Lourenco AP, Mainiero MB. Detection of mammographically occult architectural distortion on digital breast tomosynthesis screening: initial clinical experience. AJR. 2014;203:216–22.
18. Lamb LR, Bahl M, Hughes KS, Lehman CD. Pathologic upgrade rates of high-risk breast lesions on digital two-dimensional vs tomosynthesis mammography. J Am Coll Surg. 2018;226(5):858–67.
19. Shin K, Teichgraeber D, Martaindale S, Whitman GJ. Tomosynthesis-guided core biopsy of the breast: why and how to use it. J Clin Imaging Sci. 2016;8:28.
20. Mesurolle B, Brun F, Khoury ME, et al. Identification and avoidance of vessels during imaging guided biopsies: an additional role of breast tomosynthesis. Can Assoc Radiol J. 2017;68:468–70.
21. Smith A, Sumkin J, Zuley M, Chough D, Abrams G. Comparison of prone stereotactic vs. upright tomosynthesis guided vacuum assisted core breast biopsies. Radiological Society of North America 2014 Scientific Assembly and Annual Meeting, Chicago, IL. http://archive.rsna.org/2014/14003541.html. Accessed 25 Oct 2018

Chapter 4
Mammographically Guided Procedures

Romuald Ferre and Cherie M. Kuzmiak

Introduction

A stereotactic biopsy (core needle biopsy) is a minimally invasive, nonsurgical, mammographically guided, interventional breast procedure that can be performed in an outpatient setting. It is defined by the use of stereotactic images taken as a pair (+15 and −15 degrees) to calculate 3D targeting for a suspicious mammographic lesion. The procedure was developed in the 1980s. However, its clinical application became more widespread with the development and use of automated vacuum-assisted needles in the 1990s. For many medical centers, it has become the standard-of-care procedure for sampling breast lesions that are only seen mammographically.

What Is Stereotaxy?

Stereopsis is a concept that was initially described initially described by Sir Charles Wheatstone in the first half of the ninetieth century [1]. Stereopsis is the combination of two photographs of the same object taken from a different angle with a stereoscope and then viewed with a pair of lenses that displays a different picture to each eye. This allows the brain to interpret these combined two-dimensional views into a three-dimensional image [2]. When an object is seen with the eyes at the same time with two slightly different angles, two images are created (parallax). The stereopsis is achieved when the two images are fused with the visual cortex [2].

R. Ferre (✉)
Department of Radiology, Montreal General Hospital Site, McGill University, Montreal, QC, Canada

C. M. Kuzmiak
Department of Radiology, UNC School of Medicine, University of North Carolina, Chapel Hill, NC, USA

© Springer Nature Switzerland AG 2019
C. M. Kuzmiak (ed.), *Interventional Breast Procedures*,
https://doi.org/10.1007/978-3-030-13402-0_4

The principle of stereotaxy is based on the concept of stereopsis, and the process used to perform a stereotactic biopsy is nearly similar [3]. Stereotaxy is a technique of targeting that allows the determination of spatial coordinates of an object with two views that are opposed and angulated (Fig. 4.1). These two views are called paired stereotactic images. This "stereopair" is usually 15 degrees to the right and 15 degrees to the left of the 0-degree view. The 0-degree view is related to line perpendicular to image receptor, and this is called the "scout view." The "stereopair" allows the ste-

Fig. 4.1 Principles of stereotaxy. (**a**) The visualization of an object with two angulated and opposed views allows to calculate the coordinate of its spatial coordinates. Cartesian data system. (**b**) Concept of the scout view and stereotactic pair views. (**c**) An example of Cartesian coordinates

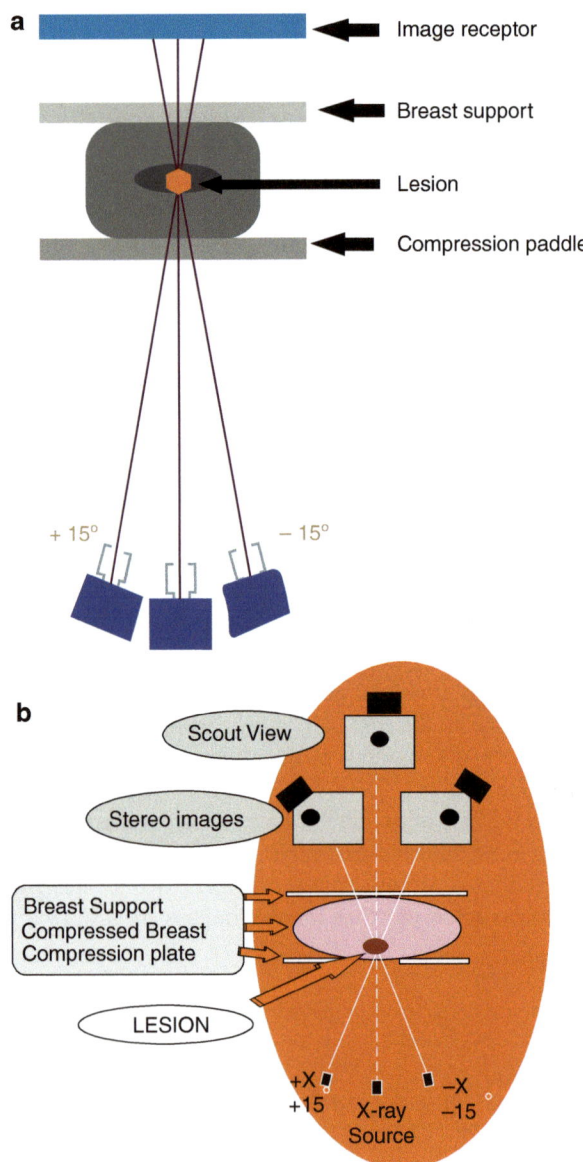

Fig. 4.1 (continued)

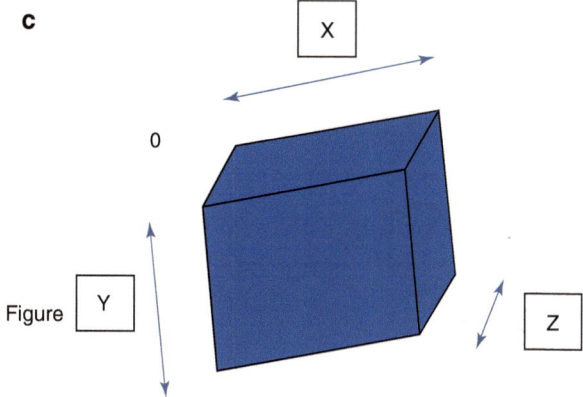

reotactic approach for a biopsy using the deviation of the parallax (incidence of position change from the observer observing an object). Parallax is the distance of apparent shift of the lesion in relation to a reference point. Computation with mathematical/geometrical tools is used to determine the coordinates, allowing to resolve lesion depth perception. Then, the computer software of the stereotactic biopsy system will determinate the accurate coordinates of the target in the three planes (trigonometry rule). Coordinates are obtained either as Cartesian (x, y, and z) or polar. Only polar coordinates allow for an angulation of the needle (alpha angle).

Breast Stereotaxy

System

Stereotaxy for the breast is designed according to the equipment/system provided [4–6]. There are two main types of system design. The first is a dedicated prone table (Fig. 4.2). For the prone table, the patient lays on her abdomen/chest, and her breast of concern will be placed through the opening on the table. The prone position favors less motion, decreases vasovagal reaction, and avoids the visualization of the biopsy equipment by the patient. The imaging equipment (CCD camera with a field of view of 5 cm × 5 cm) and biopsy device kit are positioned beneath the table with this type of design.

The second type of system allows the stereotactic-guided needle core biopsy to be performed with the patient in the seated position. These so-called "upright" biopsies are performed with a biopsy device that attaches (add-on system) to the medical site's existing mammography unit. Some of these systems may use accessories (stretcher or wedge) which allow the biopsy to be performed with the patient in a dorsal or lateral position. The advantage of this style of system design is that they are less expensive. However, women can be are at risk of increased of vasovagal reaction with this device.

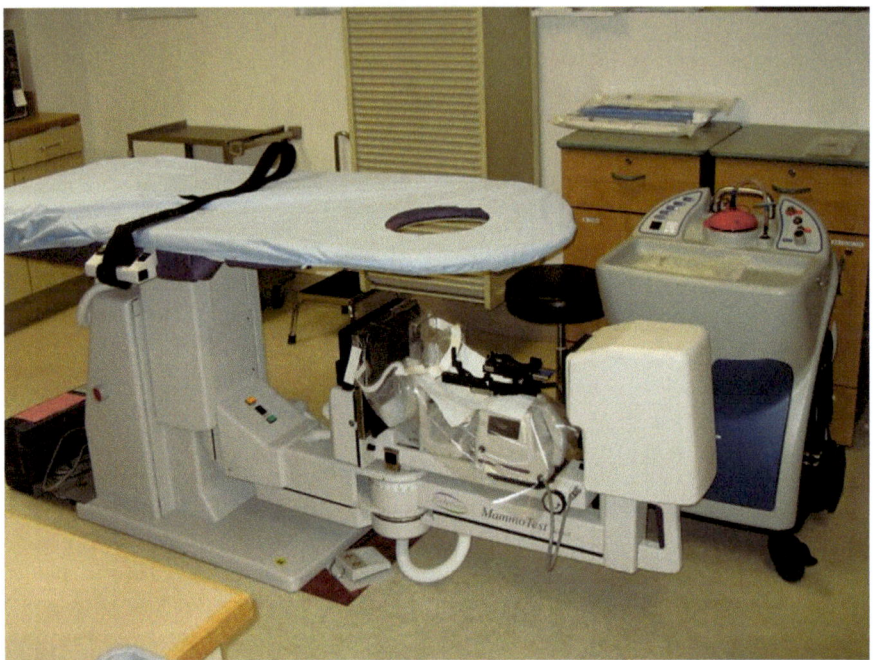

Fig. 4.2 Example of a dedicated prone stereotactic table

Biopsy Kit

A vacuum-assisted device (VAD) is the standard choice for stereotactic-guided biopsies [6–10]. The VAD is an automated needle with an internal vacuum suction that allows tissue to be pulled into the sampling chamber. VADs acquire a larger volume of tissue during lesion sampling compared to nonautomated devices. Larger sample sizes (volume) are needed to decrease the risk of under sampling. Biopsies of calcifications and areas of architectural distortion require a large sampling to minimize pathology issues [11–14].

There is diversity available for VADs. The first VAD devices were manufactured by Mammotome, which is now under Devicor Medical Products. Currently, they offer 8-gauge, 10-gauge, and 13-gauge needles depending on the biopsy system used. The EnCor breast biopsy system manufactured by SenoRX, a division of Bard Biopsy Systems, also provides a variety of needle sizes (7-gauge, 10-gauge, and 12-gauge). Hologic's ATEC breast biopsy system also has multiple different sizes (9-gauge and 12-gauge). Figure 4.3 demonstrates a selection of needle types with different gauges and aperture lengths. The different sizes and gauges of the VAD needles allow the operator flexibility to choose what is needed for optimal sampling depending on lesion location and patient's breast size.

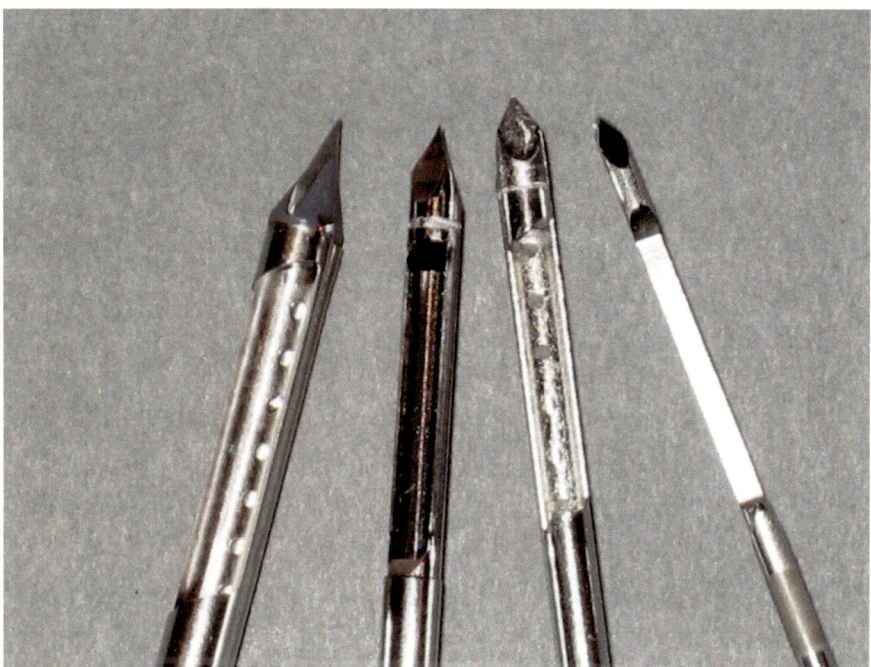

Fig. 4.3 Examples of different stereotactic core needles. There are a number of different needle gauges and designs available. The three on the left-hand side of the image are vacuum assisted

Main Indications

The main indication for stereotactic core biopsy of a BI-RADS 4 or BI-RADS 5 breast lesion is that it is not amenable to ultrasound-guided biopsy.

- Suspicious mass not seen on ultrasound
- Suspicious calcifications
- Architectural distortion not seen on ultrasound
- Focal asymmetry not seen on ultrasound

In daily practice, the majority of lesions biopsied under stereotactic guidance consist of calcifications, given the others are commonly seen on ultrasound.

Stereotactic Procedure

The biopsy procedure can be divided into three parts, as with any other image-guided procedure: the process before the biopsy, the actual biopsy, and the post-biopsy period.

Pre-biopsy

General Pre-procedural Considerations

There are several limitations related to the stereotactic core biopsy. The main one is the patient's inability to hold still during the procedure. Limitations to the prone table system include that the patient cannot lie prone for 20–30 minutes and that the patient cannot exceed the table weight limit. The table weight limit is usually 300 lbs. (up to 500 lbs. for some tables). If the patient exceeds the table weight limit, the table mechanism that raises and lowers the table could be damaged. Another limitation to the prone system is that lesions cannot be sampled from a caudal to cranial approach.

Prior to the day of the biopsy, patients should be informed there are no diet restrictions or fasting prior to this minimally invasive procedure [15–17]. Likewise, regular daily activities can be performed. Usual medications can be taken. However, some exceptions to this include blood thinners, such as Coumadin or aspirin products. These medicines should be discontinued at least 1 week prior to the biopsy to decrease the risk of bleeding and bruising. For patients on blood thinners, coordination with the patient's referring physician for best patient care is needed in case the patient cannot stop the blood thinner or needs to be switched to another medicine until the procedure is completed.

On the day of the biopsy, the technologist needs to ensure that the patient has no allergies or chance of pregnancy, if she is of childbearing age. All patients need to be informed about the biopsy process, including metallic marker clip placement at the biopsy site. Oral and written informed consent about the procedure and potential complications are required before all breast interventional procedures.

The diagnostic mammogram and any other imaging studies need to be reviewed by the radiologist. A key point is to ensure that a complete diagnostic work-up has been performed prior to the procedure. For example, CC and 90 degree lateral magnifications views have been performed to exclude the possibility of milk of calcium. Once this has been verified by the radiologist, the next step is to decide on an approach for targeting of the lesion(s) of concern. At this time, it is helpful to include the procedure technologist in the preplanning process to assist with patient positioning and equipment setup. The technologist can ensure that the appropriate equipment for the procedure is in the room. Some institutions have a preassembled biopsy kit for the day of the procedure. This may consist of syringes, needles, local anesthesia, surgical cleansing soap to disinfect skin, and sterile gloves. In addition, there should be a specimen radiography system or standard mammography equipment readily available to expedite imaging of specimen samples to decrease the patient's procedure time.

Consideration Regarding Local Anesthesia

Local anesthesia for a stereotactic core biopsy are identical to those of other radiology procedures. However, there are some specifics related to breast procedures. Namely, the breast is a low innervated organ except for the skin and nipple areolar complex. Consequently, local anesthesia must prioritize cutaneous and subcutaneous tissues regarding breast biopsies.

Lidocaine 1%, used alone or in combined with 1:100,000 epinephrine (EPI), is most commonly used as an anesthetic in breast procedures [18–20]. EPI decreases the risk of bleeding since it has vasoconstrictive action. Radiologists must be aware that there are maximal dosage amounts of these drugs and that the dose limits should not be exceeded. The maximal patient dosage of lidocaine 1% is 200 mg and for lidocaine with EPI is 500 mg [18–20]. Radiologists need to be aware that if the patient is hypovolemic or has cardiac insufficiency, these conditions may increase lidocaine concentration and lead to patient toxicity and even death. Symptoms of lidocaine overdose begin with abnormal cardiac rhythms, followed by respiratory disorders (depression and apnea) and convulsions [18–20].

All radiologists should be aware that there are contraindications to using lidocaine. These contraindications include aminosids allergies, porphyria, uncontrolled epilepsy, and a history of malignant hyperthermia. Lidocaine combined with EPI is contraindicated in patients with coronary insufficiency, ventricular arrhythmias, severe high blood pressure, hyperthyroidia, antidepressants (IMAO, trycyclique) and as an intravenous injection. Diphenhydramine is an alternative agent to those that are allergic to lidocaine [21].

There are some tips to decrease the burning feeling associated with the injection of lidocaine. One is to warm the lidocaine to body temperature before injection. Another is to add 8.4% sodium bicarbonate to buffer the lidocaine as it is supplied as a hydrochloride [22–27].

Most radiologists administer local anesthesia with a subcutaneous needle, such as a 20-gauge. After generous subcutaneous anesthesia, either the same 20-gauge or larger gauge needle can be introduced into the breast at the targeted site to provide anesthesia deeper into the breast – along the potential core needle biopsy path. Another technique that can be used to numb the tissues is called the "four cardinal points technique," i.e., injecting anesthesia at the superior, inferior, lateral, and medial aspects of the core needle entry point. In addition, current vacuum-assisted breast biopsy systems allow for the delivery of additional anesthetic during the actual biopsy/sample acquisition to minimize patient discomfort. Local anesthesia may persist for 1–2 hours after the procedure. It is important to inform the patient that she may begin to feel pain once the local anesthesia wears off.

Informed Consent

All patients need to be informed about the biopsy process. The procedure with placement of a marker clip and the potential complications of the procedure must be discussed with the patient. The patient should be made aware that the purpose of the metallic marker clip is to mark the site that was sampled. The patient should understand that the marker clip does not dissolve and that it will remain in the breast indefinitely, unless a surgeon removes it. In addition, the possibility that the lesion may not be present anymore or that it may not be able to be targeted/visualized (due to location in the breast or size) should be explained. The patient must be made aware that she will need to hold still during the entire procedure after the technologist positions her breast. It should be communicated to the patient how she will obtain her biopsy results, i.e., from her surgeon or other healthcare providers. At this time, the patient should be asked if she has any questions about the procedure and her questions answered. Afterward, both oral and written informed consent for the procedure and potential complications need to be obtained.

Positioning

The approach is one of the most important key points for stereotactic core biopsy (Fig. 4.4). The approach must be the compromise between the shortest distance from skin to lesion and the view where the lesion is the most conspicuous. The radiologist should review the imaging with the technologist to decide which approach will be the most optimal. Ideally, the approach should be the shortest distance, and the lesion is conspicuous also on that view. This interaction with the technologist facilitates the process of patient positioning and decreases the risk of repositioning the patient. Key images can be marked/annotated on the PACS (picture archiving and communication system) to help the technologist localize the target when positioning the patient's breast in the procedure compression paddle.

For the following discussion, we will use a prone table system. The patient is placed on her abdomen/chest on the table, and the breast of concern is brought through the dedicated breast opening on the table. The technologist positions the breast between the image receptor and fenestrated mammographic paddle (Fig. 4.5). Once the patient has been positioned according to the elected approach and location of the lesion in the breast, the technologist will adequately compress the breast with the paddle. During the entire procedure, the patient's breast is in mammographic compression.

A scout view x-ray of the breast in the fenestrated paddle is acquired (Fig. 4.6). The scout view is a neutral view (angle of 0 degree). This ensures that the lesion of concern is visible in the field of view (FOV). Also, the lesion should be centered in the FOV. If not, the technologist should reposition the patient/breast adequately. If the lesion is properly centered on the scout view, the procedure radiologist needs to confirm the absence of an overlapping blood vessel with the target. An overlapping blood vessel over the site of biopsy is a contraindication to performing a stereotactic biopsy since there is the risk of bleeding. The technologist can try to reposition or roll the breast tissue to move the blood vessel out of the way of the lesion. If this is not successful, targeting the lesion in the orthogonal direction may eliminate this issue. Of note, stereotactic views, which are angled, can falsely reassure that a blood vessel is out of the way of the potential core needle path.

If the lesion is centered in the FOV and no blood vessel is overlapping the lesion, stereotactic images are the next step prior to the biopsy (Fig. 4.7). Stereotactic views "stereopair" are angulated views (+15 degrees and −15 degrees). On each angulated stereotactic view, the center of the lesion is marked/targeted by the radiologist using

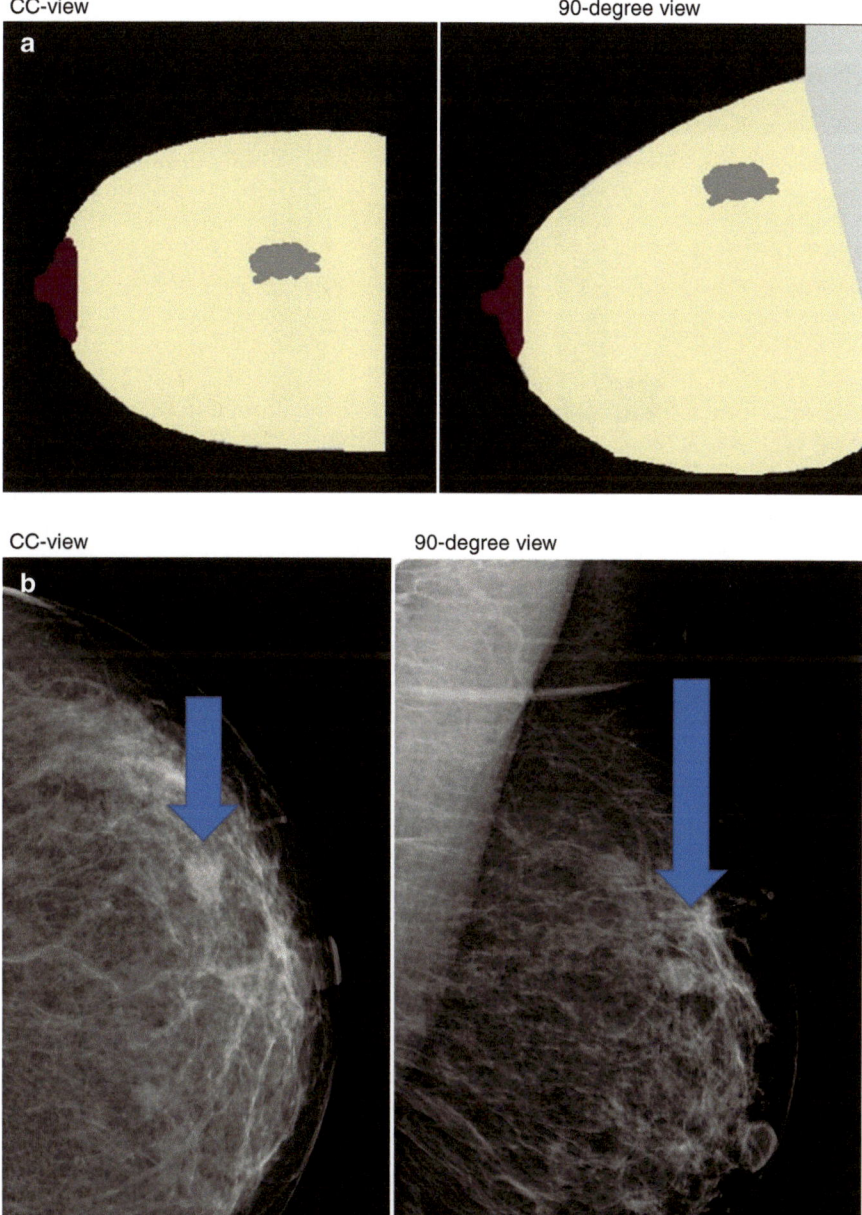

Fig. 4.4 Approach: visibility and shortest distance. (**a**) The shortest distance from the skin surface to the lesion of concern should be considered for the stereotactic core biopsy. The patient's lesion of interest is an irregular mass (dark gray) in this illustration. The shortest distance for the biopsy path would be a craniocaudal approach. (**b**) Blue arrow denotes the lesion to be sampled. The shortest distance from the skin surface to the lesion is from lateral to medial in this example

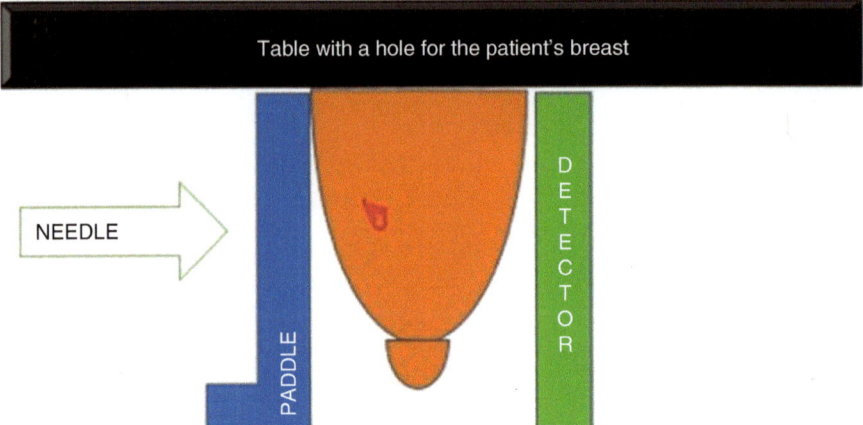

Fig. 4.5 Schematic of the patient's breast and other components of the biopsy system

computer software compatible with the stereotactic core biopsy system. At times, targeting on the superior aspect of the lesion may be warranted if the patient is likely to move. Thus, the lesion will move upward, and this target technique will anticipate this motion and change in lesion positioning.

Next, the computer software will automatically calculate the spatial coordinates. These stereotactic coordinates will either be Cartesian or polar. If the breast biopsy system uses Cartesian coordinates, the targeting information will be displayed with an x, y, and z. If the system uses polar coordinates, then the computer will display the targeting information with an h (horizontal), v (vertical), and d (depth).

After reviewing the biopsy targeting coordinates, which are reported automatically to the stereotactic device with needle guide housing, the radiologist needs to verify the computer calculated stroke margin. The "stroke margin" corresponds to the distance between the needle tip and the distance surface of the skin or the distance from the needle tip to the image receptor, depending on what stereotactic system is used. It is imperative for radiologists to know and understand the stereotactic biopsy system that they use. The stroke margin should be greater than 4 mm (or 10 mm depending on the needle and system used). If the stroke margin is negative or less than the patient safety numbers recommended by the device manufacturer, the breast can be repositioned and folded upon itself, or a second fenestrated paddle can used. The second fenestrated paddle is placed between the image receptor and the breast (the targeting fenestrated paddle is still in position). These tips can help increase breast thickness and eliminate a negative stroke margin. If these methods are not successful, then an orthogonal targeting path needs to be considered. Once safe measurements are confirmed, the biopsy needle is placed on to the housing guide, and the needle is automatically positioned to the chosen targeted location.

Fig. 4.6 Scout view. The lesion must centered within the FOV. (**a**) Schematic. (**b**) Scout view of a 2-cm mass (arrow) centered in the FOV. (**c**) The patient's breast is compressed by the paddle. The skin has been cleaned after the mass in 6b was targeted

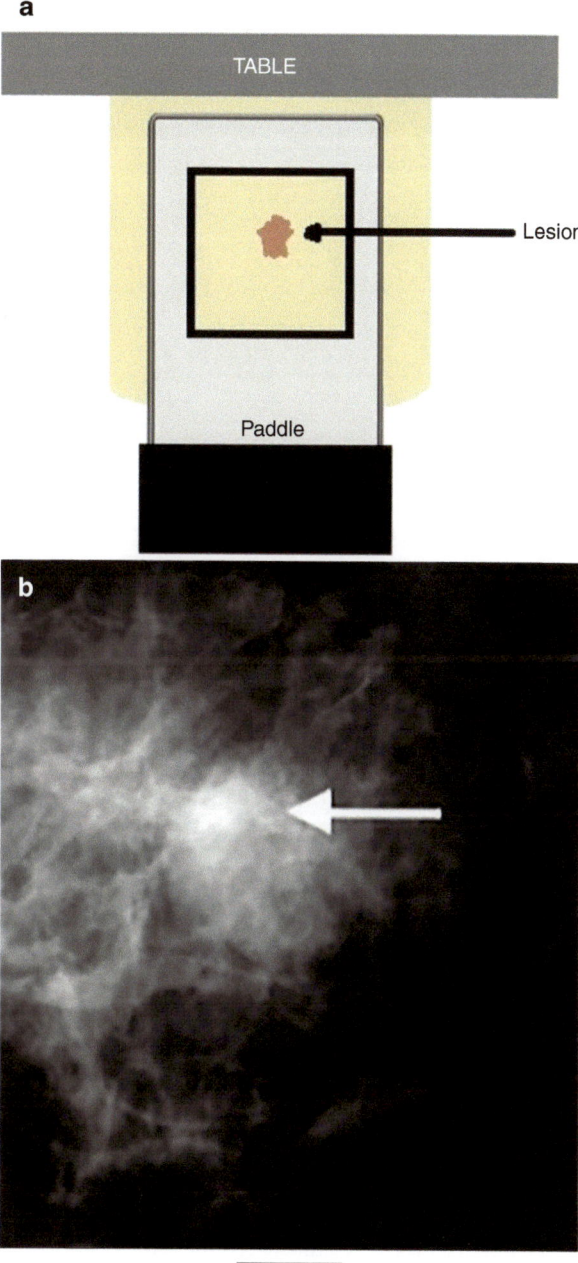

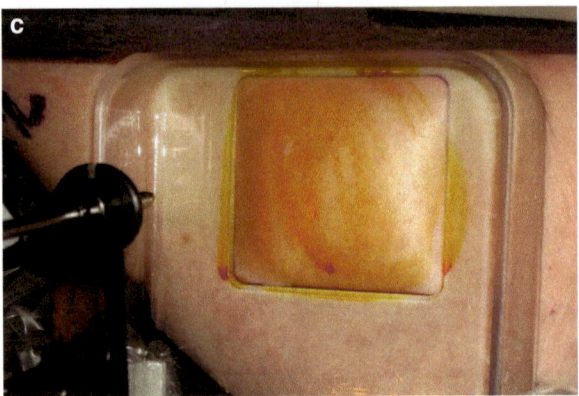

Fig. 4.6 (continued)

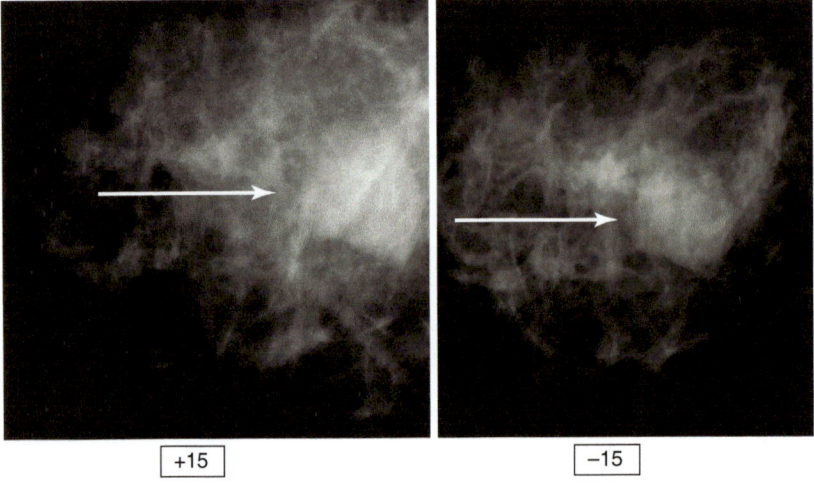

Fig. 4.7 Stereotactic views (stereopair) of a 2-cm, oval mass (arrow) that was seen on the scout view in Fig. 4.6

Biopsy Procedure

As with any biopsy, cleansing of the skin is performed with a surgical soap. The targeted skin site in the fenestrated paddle is cleaned. Afterward, it is necessary to anesthetize the skin entry point. The skin entry point is the site where the core needle biopsy will be inserted in the breast. If this not performed initially or adequately, it could create target displacement and patient discomfort. Once the site is properly numbed, a small 2–3 mm skin incision is made with a scalpel. The needle is then inserted through the small skin incision to the appropriate predetermined depth.

A "stereopair" (pre-fire images) is then acquired prior to the final advancement/firing of the needle to ensure correct needle placement. To be in appropriate position for sampling, the targeted lesion needs to be at the tip needle in both views (Fig. 4.8). If the lesion is not at the tip of the needle it both views, it has been displaced and retargeted is indicated. Once the needle is in satisfactory position, the needle is tip is advanced/fired. To minimize patient motion and repositioning, it is important to tell the patient prior to firing the needle that she will hear a loud noise and may feel a thump sensation in the breast. After the needle is fired, a tissue sample can be obtained prior to acquiring the first set of post-biopsy stereopair images. This ensures at least one core sample is obtained from the targeted site if the patient develops an immediate complication (bleeding) or wants to stop the procedure. Post-fire stereopair images are then acquired. These images will allow the radiologist to visualize needle placement in relation to the targeted lesion and if any adjustments of the needle need to be performed prior to further tissue sampling.

Traditionally, 6–12 tissue samples are obtained with a VAD from the lesion of concern. The rational to obtain 6–12 samples is to have obtained an adequate lesion sampling [28–30]. It has to be kept in mind that a small number of samples (less than 5) increase the risk of under sampling (i.e., atypical ductal hyperplasia (ADH) versus ductal carcinoma in situ (DCIS), in situ carcinoma versus invasive ductal carcinoma (IDC)) [31]. The goal of needle core biopsy is to sample the lesion, but not necessarily completely remove it with a needle. However, with stereotactic core biopsy, the lesion of concern is frequently removed, especially when it is <15 mm (Fig. 4.9). The needle device can be rotated on the needle housing with a clock roundabout approach by the radiologist to multiple different locations in the targeted lesion. Also, further dedicated sampling at a particular location can be performed by the radiologist. For example, if the lesion is located more at the 6 o'clock position relative to the sampling aperture of needle, more samples can be obtained from this location to acquire more tissue for histologic analysis. With VAD biopsy needles, vacuum suction pulls the tissue into the needle aperture, an inner needle sheath cuts the tissue (Fig. 4.10), and then the tissue sample is conveyed to an external collection chamber automatically. Since the VAD device is equipped with an aspiration system, the procedure is rarely interrupted if the patient experiences bleeding during the procedure.

Once the tissue specimens of the lesion of concern have been obtained, they should be radiographed if the lesion contained calcifications (Fig. 4.11). The specimen radiograph can be obtained on a dedicated mammography system or a dedicated specimen system ideally in the biopsy room. This important step of the procedure confirms the specimens contain calcifications and the lesion was appropriately sampled. If calcifications are note seen, more samples can be obtained from the same targeted site since the needle has not yet been removed from the patient's breast or the lesion needs to be retargeted. There is no specific need to radiograph the specimens of a non-calcified lesion.

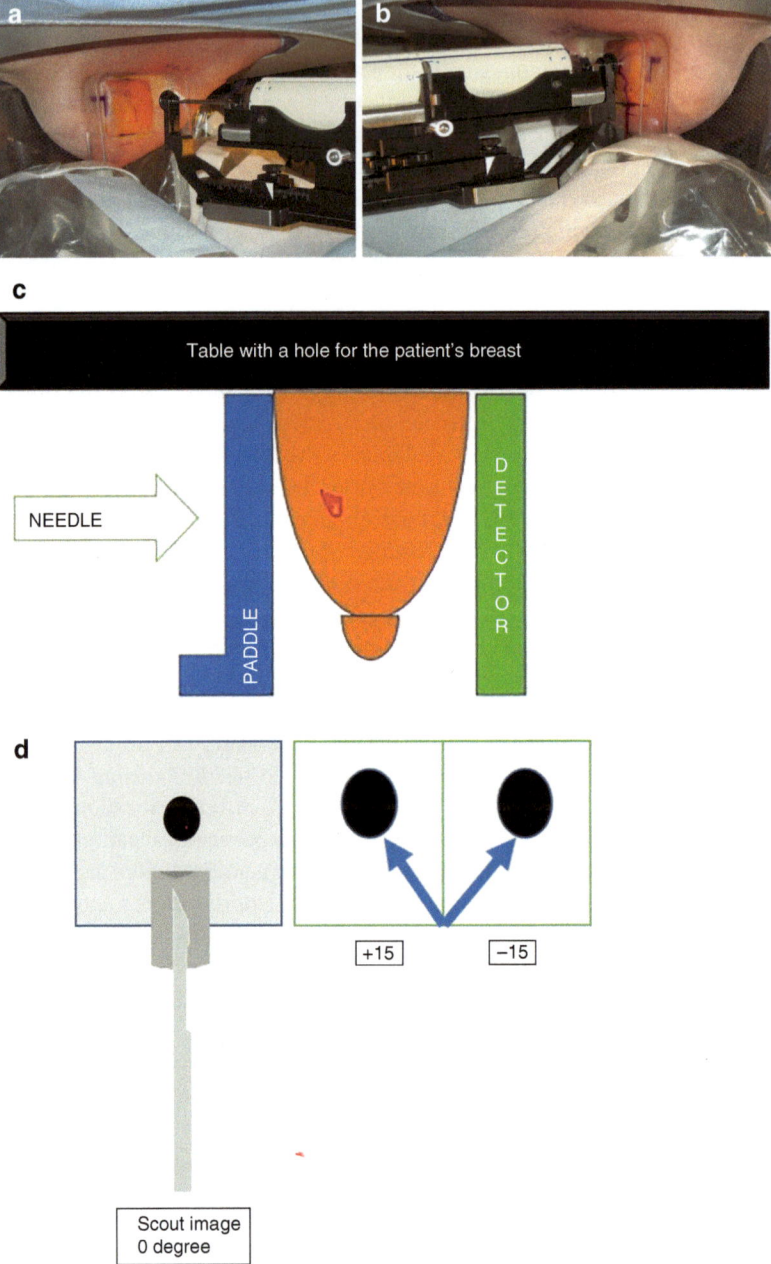

Fig. 4.8 Needle placement. (**a**) Demonstrates the needle biopsy device after targeting the lesion of concern, just prior to the tiny skin incision. (**b**) Needle device inserted and advanced into the breast at the targeted site. (**c**) Schematic of Fig. 4.8b demonstrating the positioning of the breast, needle, and lesion. (**d**) This schematic demonstrates appropriate targeting on the scout and pre-fire stereopair images. The needle tip (arrow head of the blue arrows) points directly at the lesion (black circle). (**e**) Post-fire stereopair images. These images demonstrate that the mass (arrow) was slightly displaced inferior to the needle. Therefore, appropriate sampling of the lesion would be from the 3 to 9 o'clock needle position with the great yield between the 4 and 8 o'clock areas

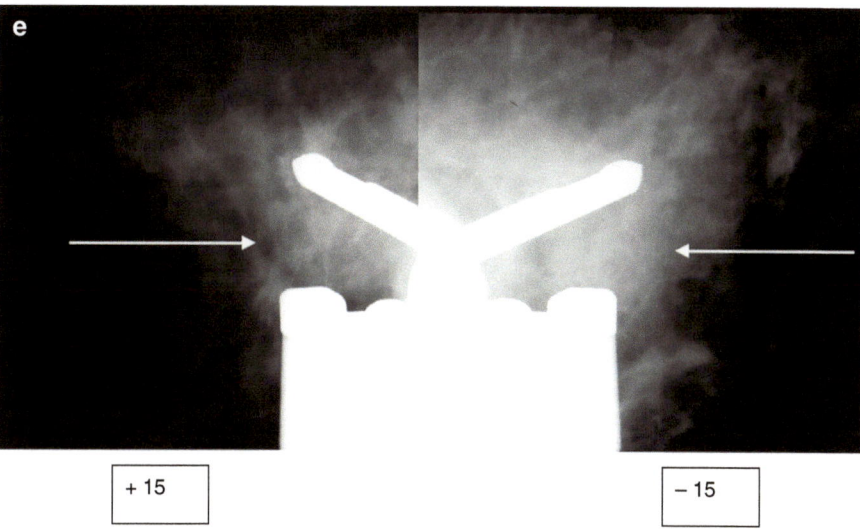

+ 15

− 15

Fig. 4.8 (continued)

Fig. 4.9 Stereotactic vacuum-assisted core biopsy. This schematic demonstrates the ability to rotate the stereotactic core needle 360 degree in the breast to sample multiple areas within a lesion

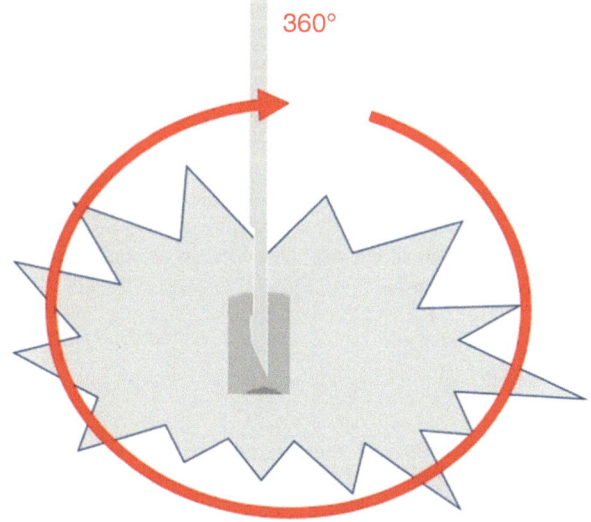

360°

If sampling of the lesion is satisfactory, a metallic marker clip is inserted via an introducer sheath into the breast. The marker clip is then deployed. There is a diversity regarding the geometric shape and deployment design of the marker clips. The purpose of the marker clip is to mark the site that was sampled. A final scout view or stereopair is acquired to confirm the marker clip was deployed (Fig. 4.12). There is a very low risk that the marker clip does not deploy. If the marker clip did not deploy, a second marker clip can be placed and confirmed prior to removal of the needle biopsy device from the breast.

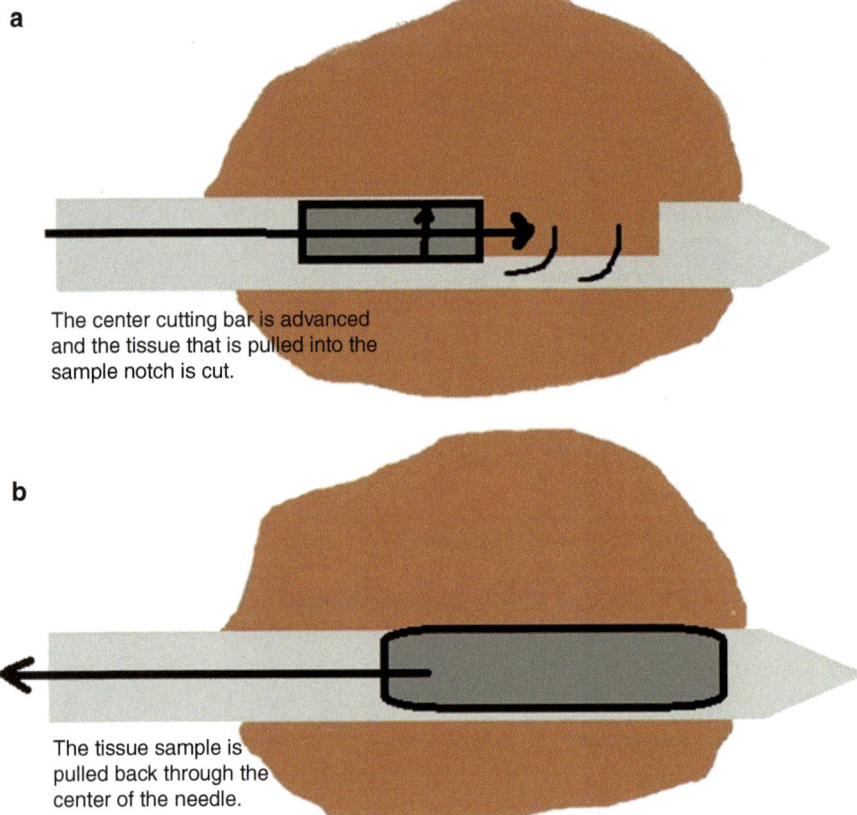

a

The center cutting bar is advanced
and the tissue that is pulled into the
sample notch is cut.

b

The tissue sample is
pulled back through the
center of the needle.

Fig. 4.10 Special features of a vacuum-assisted needle. (**a**) The rotating inner part advances forward, *cutting and capturing a sample*. The vacuum is on. (**b**) After the inner part has reached its full forward position, the notch is closed, tissue *sample is within* the inner part, and the tissue sample is pulled back through the hollow center portion of the needle

Post-Biopsy

Special care should be taken to slowly decrease the compression force of the fenestrated biopsy paddle of the patient's breast to lessen the chance that the marker clip migrates within the tissue. This phenomenon is called the "accordion effect." After removal of the needle device, the marker clip introducer, and the fenestrated paddle, manual compression is applied to the breast with sterile gauze. After hemostasis is achieved, a topical antibiotic ointment and a sterile dressing are applied to the

Fig. 4.11 A specimen radiograph of the tissue samples from a targeted lesion consisting of calcifications. Calcifications (arrows) are present in the samples

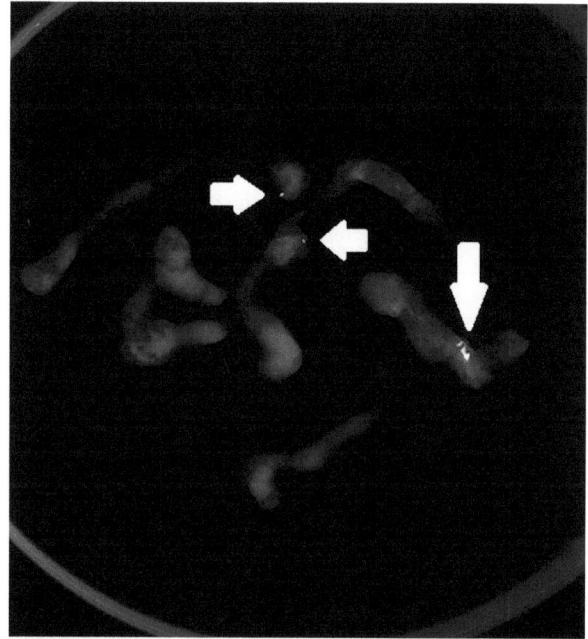

Fig. 4.12 An image from a stereopair demonstrates that the marker clip has been deployed at the biopsy site. In addition, a small amount of air from the biopsy and a small hematoma (white arrow) are also present

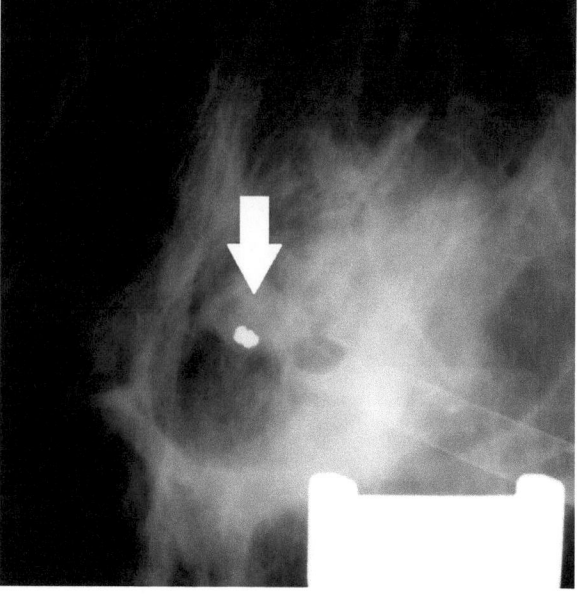

wound. The dressing consists of one of more steristrips to help with wound closure. Over the steristrip(s), a second layer of bandage consisting of a simple band aid or vinyl dressing is applied. After the biopsy site is covered with the dressing, a post-biopsy two-view (CC and 90) full-field mammogram is performed to confirm the position of the marker clip and the sampled breast lesion. This post-procedure mammogram also documents any remaining calcifications or biopsied mass components. It also confirms the appropriate lesion has been sampled.

Before the patient leaves the clinic, post-biopsy potential side effects, such as minor pain and bruising at the biopsy site, are reviewed again. A contact number in case problems arise and post-biopsy instructions are provided to the patient. Post-biopsy and wound care instructions are reviewed with the patient, and she is also provided the same information in writing. These are listed below:

- There are no diet restrictions.
- To relieve discomfort, acetaminophen (Tylenol) or ibuprofen can be taken.
- Ice can be applied to the site every 20 minutes for the first 2 hours. For example, on for 20 minutes and then let your skin warm up for 20 minutes. Then, after the 1st 2 hours, ice can be used as needed but not for more than 20 minutes at a time.
- If the ice feels too cold/stinging your skin, wrap another cloth over the ice bag to prevent damage to the skin. Ice can be used intermittently for the first 2 days if needed.
- If bleeding occurs, apply direct pressure to the site for 5–10 minutes.
- Baths, showers, hot tubs, and swimming pools are contraindicated for the first 2 days to limit the risk of infection and reduce bruising.
- Sports and any excessive activities that use of the same side arm as the biopsy are not recommended for the next 2 days to reduce bruising and bleeding.
- Leave the band aid/vinyl dressing on for 2 days. After the second day, it can be removed.
- The steristrips should be removed from the skin after 5 days.

Post-Biopsy Reporting

For any interventional breast procedure, a dictated report is needed for the patient's medical record. The report should include the following: type of biopsy performed, type of lesion biopsied and its location in the breast, the imaging method for guidance, biopsy kit/needle used, number of tissues specimens obtained, marker clip shape deployed (i.e., rod-shaped) and its location related to the biopsy site (any migration), and any patient complications. A reporting a template can be used to help simplify the dictation.

Radiology/Pathologic Correlation

Once the pathology results are available, the radiology procedure will be completed when the radiology finding and pathology are correlated. In general, the sampling success of stereotactic needle core biopsy is approximately 95% [32–34]. Most failures of this procedure are related to poor lesion visualization [32–34]. In the radiology procedure report, it should state if the radiology lesion finding and pathology are concordant/discordant and provide a management recommendation to the patient's provider/surgeon.

Concordant

If the pathology results are *benign and concordant* with the radiology findings, a follow-up mammogram is recommended to ensure interval stability. Some institutions will recommend a 1-year follow-up for all benign concordant lesions, secondary to the larger tissue samples (9-gauge) obtained for pathologic analysis with this image-guide procedure. Nevertheless, other institutions may opt for a 1-year follow-up for a specific lesion (such as a fibroadenoma) and a 6-month follow-up for non-specific benign results (fibrocystic changes or benign breast tissue). A variety of follow-up protocols exist.

When the pathology results from a needle core biopsy demonstrate a *high-risk lesion*, such as atypical ductal hyperplasia, and the imaging is *concordant and benign,* it should be stated in the report. In addition, surgical excision should be recommended and documented in the radiology report. There is a risk of histologic underestimation with atypia being upgraded to malignancy on final surgical excision [35, 36].

When the pathology results are *malignant and concordant*, the patient should follow up with a breast surgeon/breast healthcare team for further care. Additionally, if there are other imaging findings in a case with known malignancy, it should be stated in the report if additional intervention versus close follow-up is warranted. It is also valuable in these cases to confirm that the contralateral breast is negative and include that in the radiology report to help facilitate patient care.

Discordant

Pathology results are deemed *discordant with radiology findings* accounting for approximately 3–4% of cases [31, 35–37]. This is especially true when calcifications are targeted but yet are absent in the pathology analysis. In those cases, the tissue blocks can be obtained from pathology and x-rayed to help the pathologist pinpoint any calcifications for directed further tissue analysis. If no calcifications are seen on x-ray of the tissue blocks and the pathologist has exhausted the tissue block samples, further tissue sampling should be planned. This could be in the form of a second stereotactic core biopsy or an alternative would be to recommend surgical excision with preoperative localization [31, 35–37].

When a targeted lesion's imaging appearance is more worrisome than benign pathology results, it should be stated in the report that the results are *benign and discordant*. Resampling with stereotactic core biopsy or with surgical excision should be recommended. It is vital for patient care to communicate this information to the patient's provider/surgeon.

Potential Challenges

Negative Stroke Margin

This is one of the most common events during a stereotactic core biopsy (Fig. 4.13). As defined earlier, the stroke margin corresponds to the distance between the needle tip and the distance surface of the skin. However, depending on the system used, it may also represent the distance from needle tip to carbon fiber plate. Regardless of the system design, the stroke margin has to always be positive. This issue arises often into two situations: (1) the breast compresses too thin, and (2) lesion of concern is located in the immediate subareolar region of the breast. Most often these situations are remedied by switching the planned approach. The orthogonal position may allow the lesion to change sufficiently to the distal skin surface and then warrants a safe procedure. Another alternative is to inject an extra amount of local anesthesia into the superficial tissues to increase artificially the thickness of the breast. Bolstering the breast with some bandage can be a helpful technique in some situations. Compression can be applied from the nipple toward the chest wall with a wide tape, for example.

Lesion Visible One-View Only

There are cases where the lesion is only visible on one view. This can occur for architectural distortion or an asymmetry. Another example is when two lesions overlap on one view and only the orthogonal view allows one to know which lesion

Fig. 4.13 Negative stroke margin. (**a**) **Stroke margin**: distance (black arrow) from tip of needle in the fired position to the image receptor/breast support. (**b**) **Negative stroke margin**: indicates that the needle will exit the breast and strike the image receptor/breast support

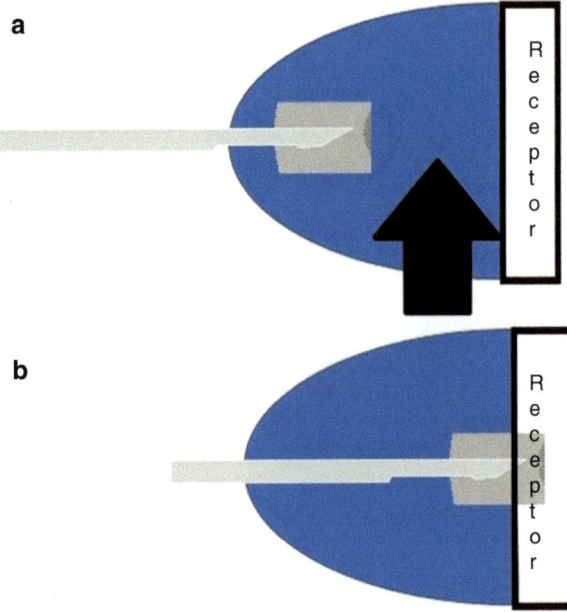

can be confidently biopsied. Tomosynthesis can be helpful to determine which approach to perform. If tomosynthesis is not available, the value of the stroke margin is an interesting parameter. If positive, this means the approach is the safe one. If negative, the approach is not the accurate one given this is the longest one.

Posterior Breast/Axillary Lesion

Posterior breast and axillary lesions may be sometimes difficult to be targeted with a stereotactic approach. An easy solution to include the patient's posterior tissue is to bring the patient's ipsilateral arm along with her breast of interest through the table aperture (Fig. 4.14). This helps to bring the lesion to be targeted into the biopsy window.

Superficial Lesion

Superficial lesions can cause many difficulties not only in targeting the lesion but also in obtaining adequate tissue samples. Superficial lesions can be very mobile and difficult for the technologist to position correctly in the FOV. These lesions can

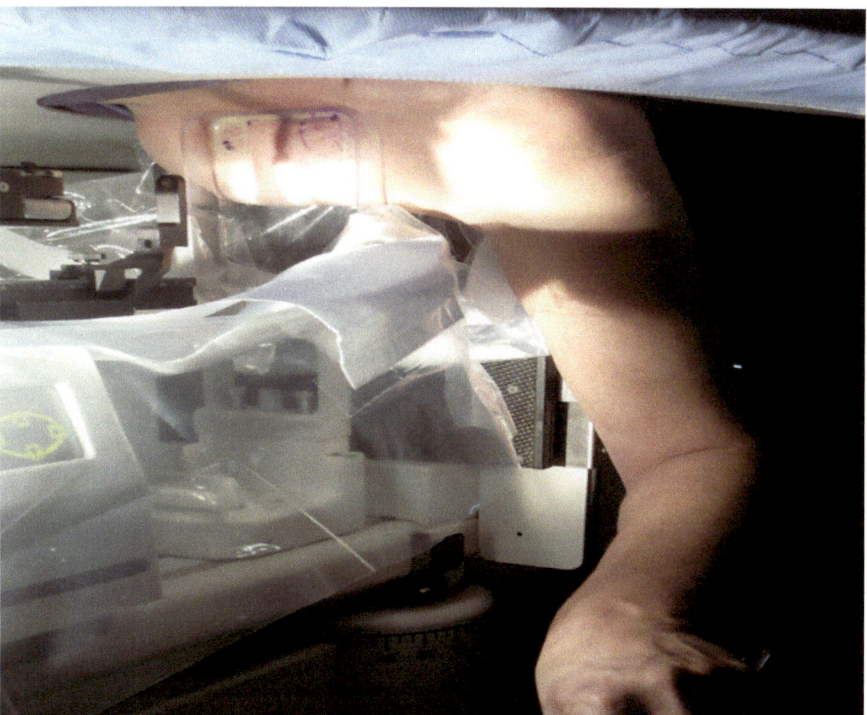

Fig. 4.14 Posterior breast/axillary lesion. The patient's arm is placed through the table aperture to allow access to far posterior breast and axillary lesions. The patient's arm is rested on a portable table

easy be displaced with local anesthesia. Additionally, there is a risk of skin breach during the biopsy given their close location to the skin. Some helpful tips include making a small skin nick and/or firing the needle outside the breast then insert slightly deeper to the lesion to protect the skin.

Retroareolar Lesion

Given to their location to the nipple areolar complex, these are often difficult to be biopsied. A retroareolar lesion is defined as lesion less than 2 centimeters from the nipple [38]. An ultrasound approach should be favored instead of stereotactic biopsy. If not, the breast should be compressed without centering on the nipple areolar complex – breast may compress too thinly. An alternative method consists of targeting the distal aspect of the lesion of concern or even supporting the anterior aspect of the breast with tape to try to increase the breast thickness.

Lesion No Longer Visible

The most common explanation is patient motion. The patient physically moved after the lesion was targeted. In order to detect patient motion during the biopsy, it may be useful to mark the skin with an ink marker inside the horizontal border of the paddle – two opposite sides of the fenestrated paddle. If the skin ink marks remain visible, the patient has not moved. If the ink marks are no longer seen, the patient has moved, and repositioning will be needed.

Local anesthesia can induce lesion displacement, especially when the lesion is superficial. Alternatively, some faint calcifications in a dense breast can be less conspicuous on the post-fire images. The needle may actually obscure them. Also, the lesions can be obscured by the local anesthesia injected into the breast or a hematoma if the patient bleeds.

Lesion Visible on One Stereopair Image

This scenario occurs when the lesion is not centered on the scout view (Fig. 4.15). If the lesion is more to the right side on the scout view, then it will not be seen on the −15-degree view. Likewise, if the lesion is more to the left side on the scout view, it will be not seen on the +15-degree view. Re-centering the lesion will eliminate this issue. However, it is possible with some systems to target the lesion using the scout view and the single stereopair image in which the lesion is seen.

Lesion No Longer Centered After Needle Advancement

It is often easier to recognize motion on the post-fire images compared to pre-fire images. Patient motion will be either the x- or y-plane. The deviation to right or left of the needle corresponds to an x-motion (Fig. 4.16). If the needle appears to the right of the lesion, then biopsy samples should be started at 6 o'clock

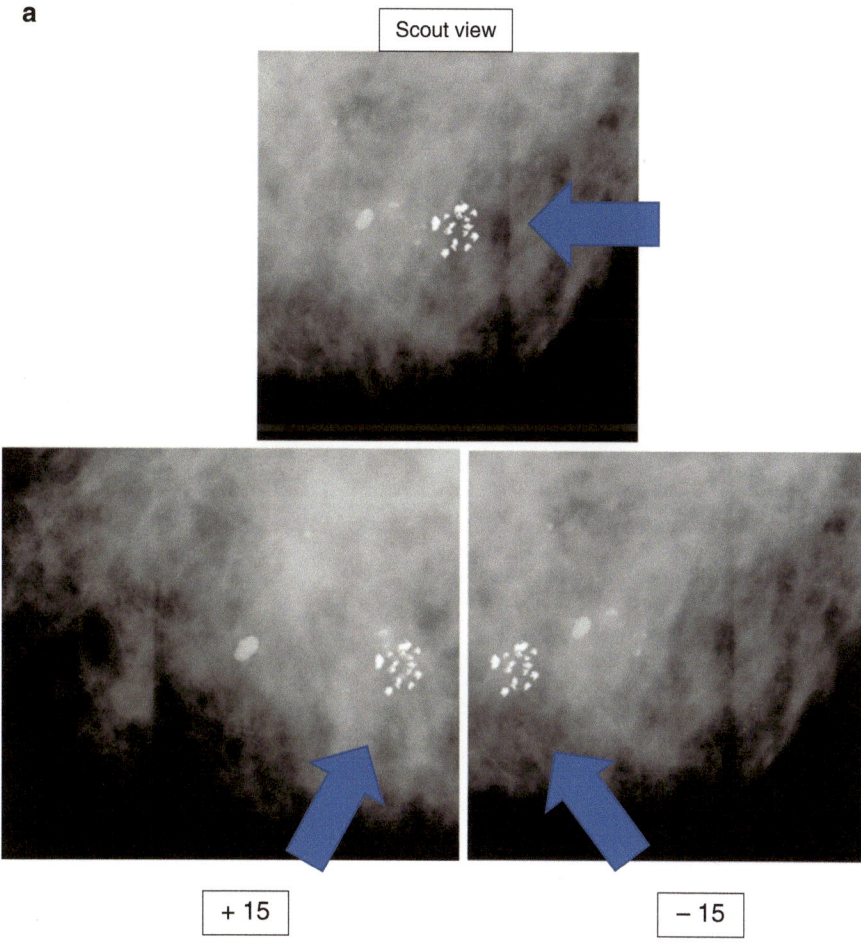

Fig. 4.15 Lesion visibility. The lesion in this example is grouped calcifications (arrow). (**a**) Example of grouped calcifications that are seen on all images. The lesion is centered on scout view and seen on the stereopair views. (**b** and **c**) Examples when the lesion is only seen on one of the stereopair images. (**b**) Illustrates the calcifications to the right of center on the scout view and are out of the FOV on the +15-degree stereo view. (**c**) Illustrates the calcifications to the left of center on the scout view and are out of the FOV on the −15-degree stereo view. Retargeting may be needed to place the lesion in the FOV on all images. However, some systems allow for targeting on the scout view and on one of the stereotactic views

b

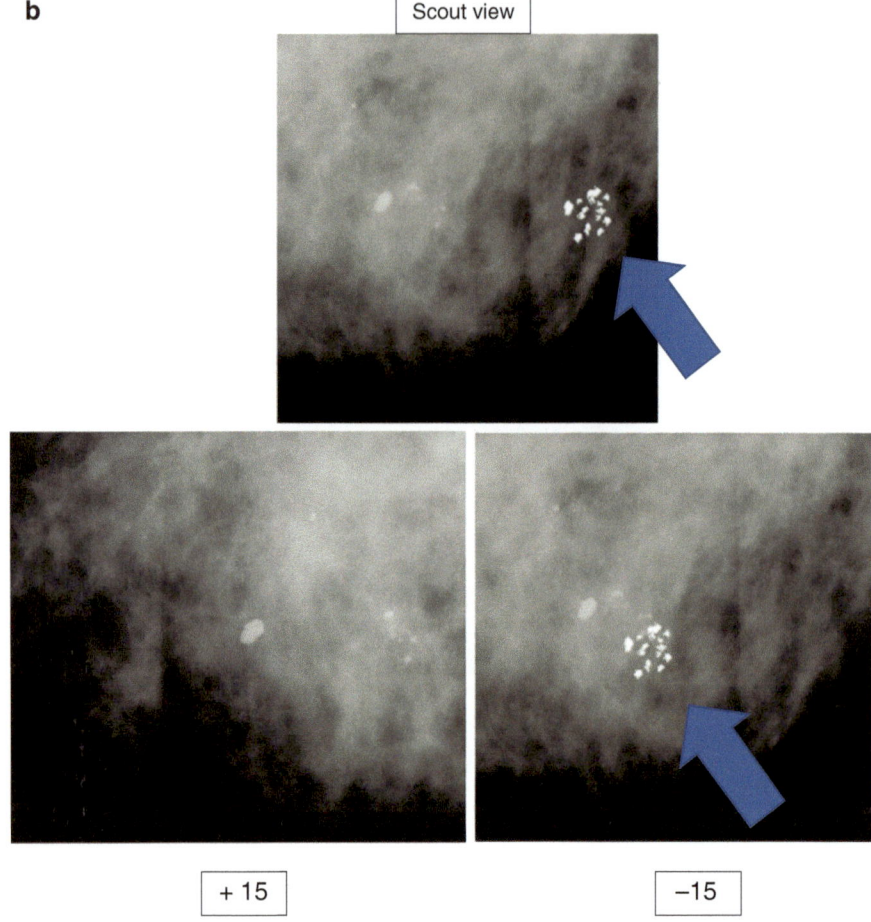

Fig. 4.15 (continued)

c

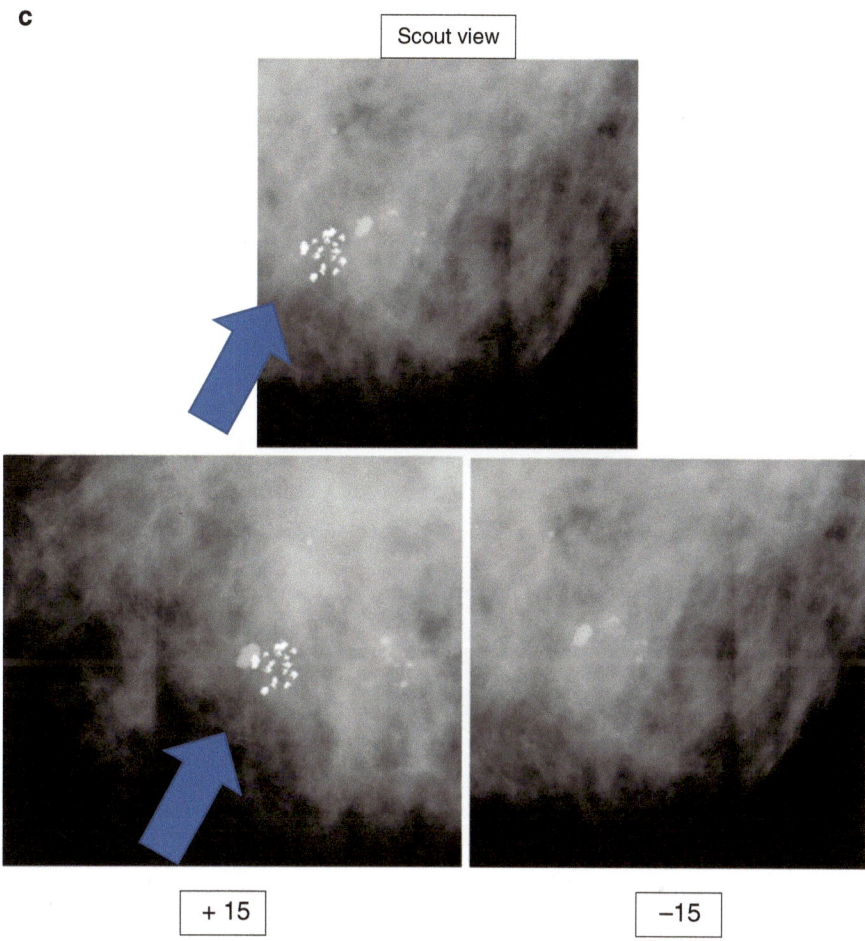

Fig. 4.15 (continued)

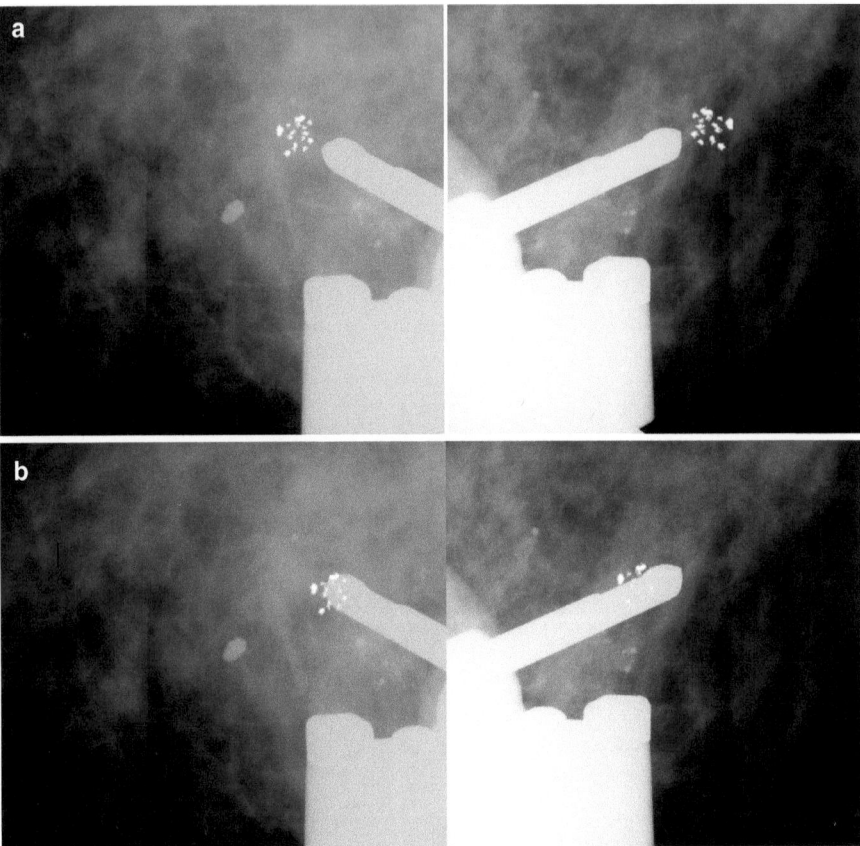

Fig. 4.16 X-plane deviation. (**a**) This is an example of no x-deviation. The needle is centered correctly on both pre-fire stereotactic pair views compared to the lesion. There is an equal projection of the tip of the needle on paired stereotactic views. (**b**) This is an example of x-deviation. The needle is not correctly centered compared to the lesion. Its tip is projected differently compared to the center of the target on the paired stereotactic views. The deviation is approximately half the distance between the tip of the needle and the center of the lesion on the most distant view. In this case, the sampling should start approximately at 6 o'clock. (**c**) Figure c represents the distance of the tip of the needle (arrow) compared to the center of the lesion (black circle). (**d**) Given the x-deviation, the needle sampling should prioritize the 6 to 12 o'clock radius positions

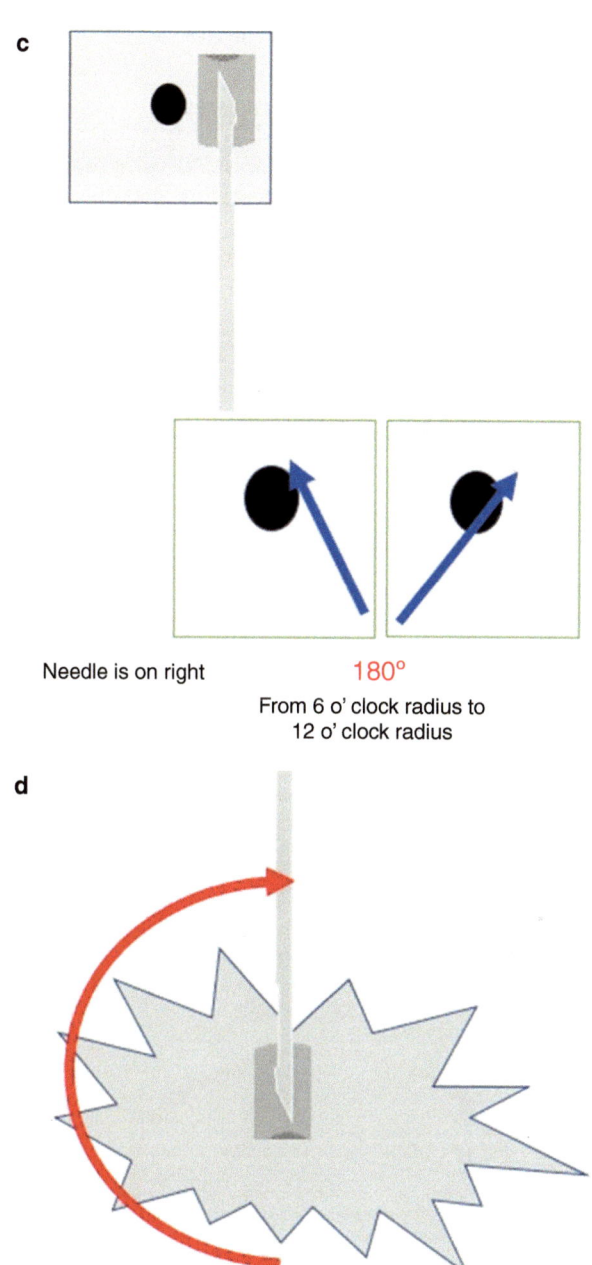

Needle is on right   180°
                          From 6 o' clock radius to
                            12 o' clock radius

Fig. 4.16 (continued)

position. If the needle appears to the left of the lesion, then biopsy samples should be started at 12 o'clock position.

Y-deviation occurs when the needle is projecting superior or inferior to the lesion (Fig. 4.17). The correction to be performed when the needle is superior to the lesion is to compress the breast inferiorly to decrease the distance between the lesion and needle. If the tip of the needle is inferior to the lesion, coordinates should be calculated manually.

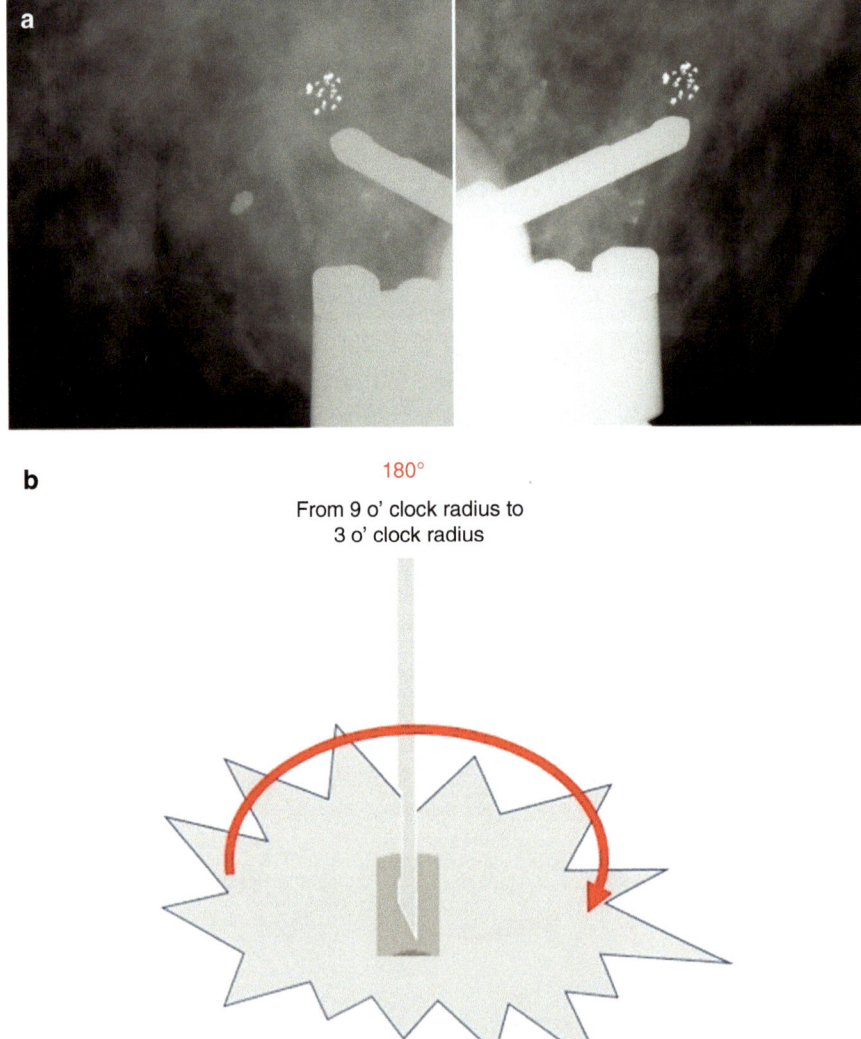

Fig. 4.17 Y-plane deviation. (**a**) The tip of the needle is located inferior to the calcifications on the pre-fire stereopair views. (**b**) Given the inferior deviation, the needle sampling should prioritize from 9 to 3 o'clock radius positions

Complications

The most common complication is bruising following a biopsy. A hematoma is defined by a 2-cm hemorrhage within the biopsy cavity [39]. Hematomas have been reported to occur in up to 11% of needle core biopsy cases [39]. A hematoma is easily visualized on post-biopsy mammograms. A reassessment with ultrasound within 1 week could be performed, especially in cases of patient discomfort. If the hematoma is symptomatic or it continues to increase in size, an aspiration under ultrasound guidance could be offered to the patient.

Uncontrolled bleeding is the worst-case scenario. This is estimated to occur in 0.1% of cases [39]. This may lead to emergency surgery to control the bleeding. This risk can be decreased by avoiding biopsy of vascular calcifications or adjacent vessels. Identifying the post-biopsy needle track in the breast with ultrasound using color Doppler may allow for better direct compression to achieve hemostasis if manual compression fails.

Infection is a rare complication, 0.1% of cases [39]. This is often due to patient comorbidities or non-compliance to wound care instructions. Implant rupture is an exceptional case of complication. Patients with breast implants must be informed prior to the biopsy of this particular risk.

Marker clip migration is another associated complication of this procedure, and it occurs in approximately 21% of cases [40]. Clip migration is defined by a > 2-cm displacement of the clip marker from the targeted site [40]. The marker clip can be located superficially or deep to target along biopsy track. Marker clip migration is more common in fatty breasts [40].

Summary/Conclusion

Stereotactic-guided percutaneous breast biopsy is an accurate, efficient, and cost-effective method of sampling breast abnormalities. This minimally invasive procedure is simple to perform and is well tolerated by patients. Its underestimation of disease/false-negative rate is less than other types of image-guided biopsy systems and can be attributed to the use of large gauge vacuum-assisted needles that obtain robust histologic samples for pathologic evaluation. It should be noted that this procedure is not curative of malignant results. As with any other image-guided procedure, a stereotactic needle core biopsy requires careful attention by the radiologist during the entire biopsy process for an optimal sampling. Radiology/pathologic correlation is mandatory and directly impacts patient management. Lastly, multidisciplinary collaboration and communication are key for diagnostic success and improved patient care.

Needle Localization

Abstract
Preoperative needle localization is an increasingly popular technique used to guide/mark a breast lesion for surgical removal. There are several devices used

for lesion localization. This section provides a review of the procedure, tips for success, and future developments.

Introduction

Breast cancer screening has resulted in increased detection of non-palpable breast cancer. The development and implementation of wire localization for non-palpable breast lesions began in the 1970s, and it continues to be used in daily clinical practice [41]. All current needle localization devices for breast lesions have a similar design: a guiding needle containing a metallic wire for targeting with the needle caliber ranging from 18- to 21-gauge. There are a variety of needle and wire lengths available allowing the radiologist to adjust for the size of the patient's breast/volume and the location of the lesion(s) to be targeted. Two parameters are essential for the procedure: the wire rigidity and its tip/hook design. The wire must be stiff enough to limit the risk of kinking/bending with insertion into the breast and transection during surgery. In addition, the distal aspect of the wire has to remain in position after deployment at the targeted site. There is the potential risk of wire displacement/migration within a fatty breast and with long operative times due to the lack of the distal aspect of the wire to firmly anchor in the tissue [42]. The most common localizing needle wire devices are either a rigid needle system with a distal J-curved wire tip (J-wire) in which the system is entirely placed and left in the breast for localization or a hook wire system in which the needle is removed from the breast after wire deployment.

Main Indications

The main indications are the following:

- Breast lesion for which surgical excision is recommended.
    - Definitive surgery for breast cancer
    - Discordant radiology and pathology results after needle core biopsy
    - High-risk lesion diagnosed on needle core biopsy, such as atypical ductal hyperplasia
- Lesion(s) not amenable to needle core biopsy.

Procedure

Pre-planning

As in any procedure, the diagnostic mammogram and any other imaging studies need to be reviewed by the radiologist. It is also helpful to include the technologist that will be assisting with the procedure in this step in order to optimize patient care and clinical workflow. If the lesion of concern is visible on mammography only, the lesion should be targeted for localization prior to surgery. If the lesion is no longer visible after a needle core biopsy, then the marker clip that was placed at the time of the needle core biopsy should be targeted. Of note, there will be cases in which the lesion is no longer visible from a prior biopsy and/or the marker clip has migrated from the biopsied site. In these cases, then the tissue site (as seen on the pre-biopsy mammogram) of the prior biopsied lesion should be localized. It is also important to discuss these cases with the patient's surgeon. In cases of extensive lesions, in which breast conservation surgery is appropriate, bracketing should be considered [42]. Bracketing consists of targeting the posterior and anterior aspect of the lesion(s). The majority of the time, this can be performed with two wires. However, there may be cases in which more than two wires are needed for targeting to help guide the surgeon intraoperatively.

Once this step is performed, the approach of the localization is determined by the shortest distance between the lesion(s) and the skin surface. If needed, the distance can be compared between the orthogonal, craniocaudal (CC), and ninety-degree (90°) views. However, if the lesion is poorly visualized for targeting using the shortest approach, then the orthogonal approach, which may be longer, can be used for localization guidance. This information can be marked on a key image prior to the procedure to assist the technologist to determine the approach. This information will also help facilitate positioning of the patient at the start of the procedure. Once the approach is chosen, the next step is to select an appropriate needle length. This can be done by measuring the distance from the skin surface to the lesion/marker clip on the pre- or post-biopsy mammogram. In cases where a lesion is the borderline in distance between two needle lengths, it may be more convenient to have a longer needle available for use. For example, the lesion measures 5.5 cm from the skin surface, and the radiologist has both 5-cm and 7-cm needle lengths available. It may be more helpful to use the 7-cm-length needle – better to be too long than too short.

Procedure

After the procedure and risks are explained to the patient, both oral and written consent must be obtained. If the patient is unable to give consent, consent needs to be obtained from the patient's guardian or power of attorney. Afterward, the patient is positioned – preferably in the seated position in a chair – and the breast of concern is compressed with a specific mammographic paddle (fenestrated alphanumeric grid) against the skin entry point. A scout view of the breast is then obtained (Fig. 4.18). During this time, the patient remains in compression, while the image is reviewed by the radiologist. It can be helpful if the technologist marks the patient's skin with an ink marker along the inside edges of the grid to evaluate any patient movement that may potentiate repositioning and retargeting at the onset of the procedure. Once the target is confirmed in the FOV of the alphanumeric grid, the skin of the breast inside the grid is cleansed with an institutional approval, topical surgical product. The

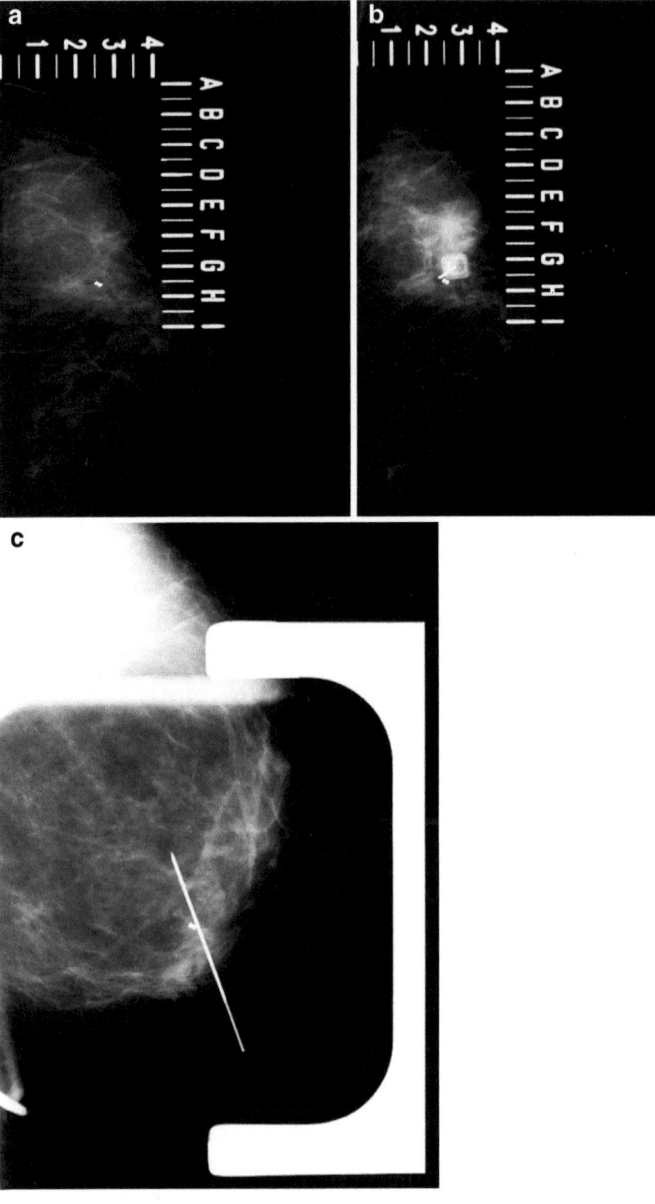

Fig. 4.18 This 48-year-old patient underwent a stereotactic core biopsy for grouped calcifications in the left breast 6 o'clock position with marker clip placement. The calcifications were removed on the stereotactic core biopsy (not shown), and a dumbbell-shaped marker clip was deployed at the biopsy site. Needle core biopsy pathology demonstrated atypical ductal hyperplasia with associated calcifications. The patient then underwent preoperative wire localization under mammographic guidance. Final surgical pathology demonstrated atypical ductal hyperplasia without carcinoma. Mammographic needle localization. (**a**) CC view with alphanumeric grid. (**b**) CC view with alphanumeric grid and needle placed. (**c**) 90-degree orthogonal view with depth of needle visualization. (**d**) CC and 90-degree views post wire placement with metallic bbs on the nipple and the skin surface of the wire entrance. (**e**) Specimen radiograph demonstrating the surgically excised marker clip and intact localization wire

CC-View   90-View

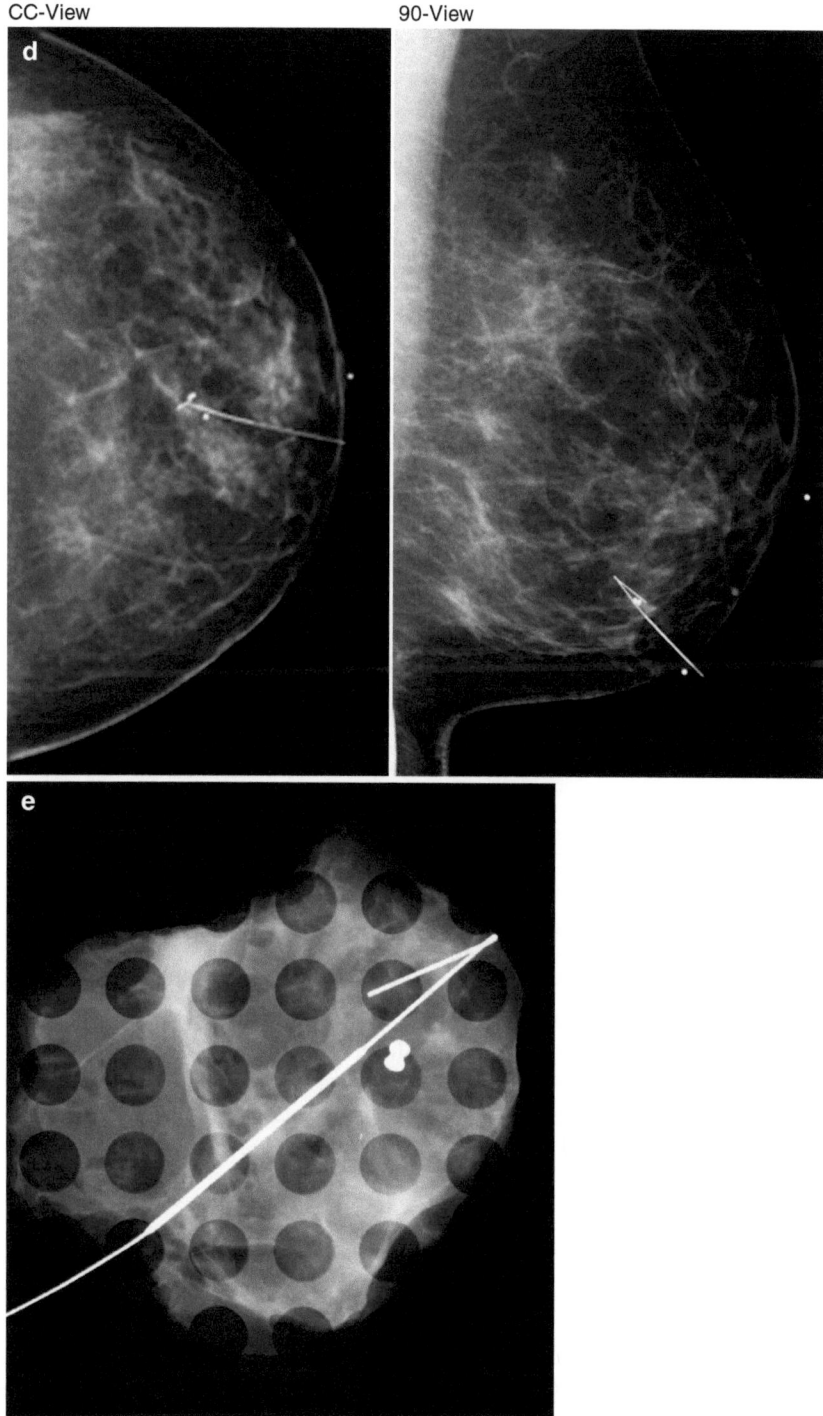

Fig. 4.18 (continued)

lesion coordinates (i.e., C, 4) are chosen by the radiologist, and local anesthesia of the skin and deep breast tissue at this site are performed, usually with lidocaine 1%. Once local anesthesia is achieved, the localization needle is placed and advanced along the needle path aided by a light source. It is important during placement of the needle that the shadow of the needle hub superimposes directly on skin entry point to ensure that the needle does not deviate from the target.

Targeting can be performed with two methods:

- *Alphanumeric coordinates*: Once the needle is positioned at the appropriate location, an orthogonal view is required to ensure the needle at the correct depth. Consequently, the breast is uncompressed, and patient will be gently repositioned in the orthogonal view.
- *Stereotactic views*. This technique can be faster given the stereotactic approach allows all three coordinates on the initial scout view. This limits the risk of needle migration when repositioning the patient.

Orthogonal images are then obtained to confirm needle placement. If the needle tip is at the appropriate localization in relation to the targeted lesion/marker clip, the wire is deployed. With the rigid needle system, the distal J-curved wire tip is advanced, and the entire device is left in place. When using a hook wire system, the wire is threaded through the hollow of the needle. The wire is advanced through the needle until the burnish mark on the wire and hub of the needle are approximated. Then, the wire is held firmly, and the needle is removed from the breast. Thus, only the wire remains in the breast marking the lesion/site.

Post-Procedure

Once the needle localization is complete and the wire(s) is/are deployed, a post-procedure mammogram is acquired for wire documentation and for surgical guidance. The post-procedure mammogram consists of two orthogonal views, most commonly a CC and 90. A metallic BB can be placed on the nipple and at the skin site of the wire(s). This will allow easier visualization of important landmarks for surgical planning. The criteria of success of needle localization are when the hook wire/tip is located less than 1 cm from the lesion or clip marker [43]. A post-procedure diagram can help summarize the wire position relatively to the target for the surgeon.

Helpful Tips

- The J-wire localization system allows for repositioning; however, the hook wire system does not once the wire is deployed.
- It may be helpful to deploy the needle/wire device just slightly deeper than the target. This can minimize the likelihood of the device/wire being pulled out or it being placed too shallow (accordion effect from the mammographic paddle).

- In challenging cases or if there is any uncertainty of the needle position, additional views should be performed. This includes magnification views to confirm needle/wire targeting or confirmation of placement, i.e., difficult to visualize calcifications.
- For posterior lesions (adjacent to the pectoralis muscle), the needle/wire can be deployed anterior (<1 cm) to the lesion, i.e., the lesion is located between the localization device and the muscle. The pectoralis muscle/pectoralis fascia will be the posterior surgical boundary.
- For anterior/retroareolar lesions, the needle/wire can be placed posterior (<1 cm) to the lesion to ensure surgical removal.
- For superficial lesions, the needle/wire can be inserted slightly deeper than the lesion to minimize the risk when the needle/wire gets pulled out.
- If the needle localization appears in a non-satisfactory position relative to the targeted lesion(s), it is preferable to repeat the procedure and deploy another wire to ensure optimal surgical removal of the lesion(s).
- If the lesion or marker clip is visible under ultrasound, ultrasound-guided preoperative needle localization is preferable since the procedure is faster and more comfortable for the patient.

Complications

The most common complication of this procedure is a vasovagal reaction. Other complications include hemorrhage, infection, and rarely a retained wire fragment from surgical transection.

Surgical Specimen

An x-ray of the surgical specimen should be performed to document removal of the targeted lesion, marker clip, and intact localization wire [44]. If one of the localized findings or devices is not present in the specimen radiograph, the surgeon should be notified immediately, and given guidance to which direction, more tissue should be excised to ensure removal of the lesion, marker clip, or wire.

Localization Advances

Preoperative needle/wire localization has been the gold standard for the last several decades to provide guidance to our surgical colleagues in removing non-palpable breast lesions. However, there are disadvantages with this system. These disadvantages include patient discomfort, wire migration, non-ideal wire entry point for the surgical approach, and inefficient surgical scheduling since the needle localization procedure is conventionally performed the same day as the surgery [45]. To overcome these obstacles, both radioactive and non-radioactive localization seeds/reflectors have been developed [45]. We refer the reader to the ultrasound-guided breast procedure chapter in this book for further reading about these specific devices. Mammographic-guided, preoperative localization of a breast lesion/marker clip with these new devices uses the same steps as with a traditional needle localization. However, instead of deploying a needle/wire, a pre-loaded introducer needle is used to deploy the seed/reflector to the breast. We anticipate continued clinical acceptance and further use of these products.

References

1. Wheatstone C, Dufour PT. Contribution à la physiologie de la vision. Tr. de l'anglais, complété par des conseils pratiques et des planches d'exercices pour faciliter la vue à l'œil nu du relief des clichés stéréoscopiques, par Pierre Th. Dufour. Lausanne, La Concorde, 1919.
2. Nam KW, Park J, Kim IY, Kim KG. Application of stereo-imaging technology to medical field. Healthc Inform Res. 2012;18:158–63.
3. Bolmgren J, Jacobson B, Nordenström B. Stereotaxic instrument for needle biopsy of the mamma. AJR Am J Roentgenol. 1977;129(1):121–5.
4. Azavedo E, Svane G, Auer G. Stereotactic fine-needle biopsy in 2594 mammographically detected non-palpable lesions. Lancet. 1989;1(8646):1033–6.
5. Parker SH, et al. Stereotactic breast biopsy with a biopsy gun. Radiology. 1990;176:741–7.
6. Doyle AJ, et al. Decubitus stereotactic core biopsy of the breast: technique and experience. AJR Am J Roentgenol. 1999;172:688–90.
7. Burbank F, Parker SH, Fogarty TJ. Stereotactic breast biopsy: improved tissue harvesting with the Mammotome. Am Surg. 1996;62(9):738–44.
8. Kettritz U, Rotter K, Schreer I, Murauer M, Schulz-Wendtland R, Peter D, Heywang-Köbrunner SH. Stereotactic vacuum-assisted breast biopsy in 2874 patients: a multicenter study. Cancer. 2004;100(2):245–51.
9. Lourenco AP, Mainiero MB, Lazarus E, Giri D, Schepps B. Stereotactic breast biopsy: comparison of histologic underestimation rates with 11- and 9-gauge vacuum-assisted breast biopsy. AJR Am J Roentgenol. 2007;189(5):W275–9.
10. Hahn M, Okamgba S, Scheler P, Freidel K, Hoffmann G, Kraemer B, Wallwiener D, Krainick-Strobel U. Vacuum-assisted breast biopsy: a comparison of 11-gauge and 8-gauge needles in benign breast disease. World J Surg Oncol. 2008;6:51.
11. Bassett L, Winchester DP, Caplan RB, et al. Stereotactic core-needle biopsy of the breast: a report of the joint task force of the American College of Radiology, American College of Surgeons, and College of American Pathologists. CA Cancer J Clin. 1997;47(3):171–90.
12. Liberman L. Centennial dissertation. Percutaneous imaging-guided core breast biopsy: state of the art at the millennium. AJR Am J Roentgenol. 2000;174(5):1191–9.
13. White RR, Halperin TJ, Olson JA Jr, Soo MS, Bentley RC, Seigler HF. Impact of core-needle breast biopsy on the surgical management of mammographic abnormalities. Ann Surg. 2001;233(6):769–77.
14. Kaufman CS, Delbecq R, Jacobson L. Excising the re-excision: stereotactic core-needle biopsy decreases need for re-excision of breast cancer. World J Surg. 1998;22(10):1023–7; discussion 1028.

15. Parker SH, Klaus AJ. Performing a breast biopsy with a directional, vacuum-assisted biopsy instrument. Radiographics. 1997;17(5):1233–52.
16. Canadian Association or Radiologist (2004), X-ray guided (stereotactic) breast biopsy. Retrieved 27 January 2010, from Radiology for patients web-site: http://www.radiologyinfo.ca
17. Somerville P, Seifert PJ, Destounis SV, Murphy PF, Young W. Anticoagulation and bleeding risk after core needle biopsy. AJR Am J Roentgenol. 2008;191(4):1194–7.
18. Ottawa Regional Women's Breast Health Centre, Stereotactic Guided Breast Core Biopsy (Brochure). Author Unknown, 2003.
19. Novy DM, Price M, Hunyh PT, Schuetz A. Percutaneous core biopsy of the breast: correlates of anxiety. Acad Radiol. 2001;8:467–72.
20. Martin S, Jones JS, Wynn BN. Does warming local anesthetic reduce the pain of subcutaneous injection? Am J Emerg Med. 1996;14:10–2.
21. Colaric KB, Overton DT, Moore K. Pain reduction in lidocaine administration through buffering and warming. Am J Emerg Med. 1998;16:353–6.
22. Pavlidakey PG, Brodell EE, Helms SE. Diphenhydramine as an alternative local anesthetic agent. J Clin Aesthet Dermatol. 2009;2(10):37–40.
23. Cragg AH, Berbaum K, Smith TP. A prospective blinded trial of warm and cold lidocaine for intra-dermal injection. AJR Am J Roentgenol. 1988;150:1183–4.
24. Klein EJ, Shugerman RP, Leigh-Taylor K, et al. Buffered lidocaine: analgesia for intravenous line placement in children. Pediatrics. 1995;95:709–12.
25. Luhmann J, Hurt S, Shootman M, Kennedy R. A comparison of buffered lidocaine versus ELA-max before peripheral intravenous catheter insertions in children. Pediatrics. 2004;113(3):217–20.
26. Matsumoto AH, Reifsnyder AC, Hartwell GD, et al. Reducing the discomfort of lidocaine administration through pH buffering. J Vasc Interv Radiol. 1994;5:171–5.
27. Zagouri F, Sergentanis T, Gounaris A, et al. Pain in different methods of breast biopsy: emphasis on vacuum-assisted breast biopsy. Breast. 2008;17:71–5.
28. Penco S, Rizzo S, Bozzini AC, et al. Stereotactic vacuum-assisted breast biopsy is not a therapeutic procedure even when all mammographically found calcifications are removed: analysis of 4,086 procedures. AJR Am J Roentgenol. 2010;195:1255–60.
29. Liberman L, Kaplan JB, Morris EA, et al. To excise or to sample the mammographic target: what is the goal of stereotactic 11-gauge vacuum-assisted breast biopsy? AJR Am J Roentgenol. 2002;179:679–83.
30. Margolin FR, Kaufman L, Jacobs RP, et al. Stereotactic core breast biopsy of malignant calcifications: diagnostic yield of cores with and cores without calcifications on specimen radiographs. Radiology. 2004;233:251–4.
31. Burbank F. Stereotactic breast biopsy of atypical ductal hyperplasia and ductal carcinoma in situ lesions: improved accuracy with directional, vacuum-assisted biopsy. Radiology. 1997;202(3):843–7.
32. Parker SH, Burbank F, Jackman RJ, et al. Percutaneous large-core breast biopsy: a multi-institutional study. Radiology. 1994;193(2):359–64.
33. Brenner RJ, Bassett LW, Fajardo LL, et al. Stereotactic core-needle breast biopsy: a multi-institutional prospective trial. Radiology. 2001;218(3):866–72.
34. Parker SH, Burbank F. A practical approach to minimally invasive breast biopsy. Radiology. 1996;200(1):11–20.
35. Smith DN, Christian RL, Meyer JE. Large-core needle biopsy of nonpalpable breast cancers: the impact on subsequent surgical excisions. Arch Surg. 1997;132(3):256–9; discussion 260.
36. Jackman RJ, Nowels KW, Rodriguez-Soto J, Marzoni FA Jr, Finkelstein SI, Shepard MJ. Stereotactic, automated, large-core needle biopsy of nonpalpable breast lesions: false-negative and histologic underestimation rates after long-term follow-up. Radiology. 1999;210(3):799–805.

37. Lee CH, Philpotts LE, Horvath LJ, Tocino I. Follow-up of breast lesions diagnosed as benign with stereotactic core-needle biopsy: frequency of mammographic change and false-negative rate. Radiology. 1999;212(1):189–94.
38. Giess CS, Keating DM, Osborne MP, et al. Retroareolar breast carcinoma: clinical, imaging, and histopathologic features. Radiology. 1998;207:669–73.
39. Berg W, Yang WT. Diagnostic imaging breast. 2nd edn. Amirsys; 2013, Chapters 10–20.
40. Kass R, et al. Clip migration in stereotactic biopsy. Am J Surg. 2002;184(4):325–31.
41. Hall FM, Kopans DB, Sadowsky NL, Homer MJ. Development of wire localization for occult breast lesions: Boston remembers. Radiology. 2013;268(3):622–7.
42. Liberman L, Kaplan J, Van Zee K, Morris EA, LaTrenta L, et al. Bracketing wires for preoperative breast needle localization. AJR. 2001;177:565–72.
43. Chadwick DR, Shorthouse AJ. Wire-directed localization biopsy of the breast: an audit of results and analysis of factors influencing therapeutic value in the treatment of breast cancer. Eur J Surg Oncol. 1997;23(4):128–33.
44. Rubin E, Simpson JF. Breast specimen radiography: needle localization and radiographic pathologic correlation. Philadelphia: Lippincott-Raven; 1998.
45. Mango VL, Wynn RT, Feldman S, Friedlander L, Desperito E, Patel SN, et al. Beyond wires and seeds: reflector-guided breast lesion localization and excision. Radiology. 2017;284(2):365–71.

Chapter 5
MRI-Guided Biopsy Procedures

Jean M. Seely

Introduction

Breast MRI has become essential to clinical breast imaging practice in the past 20 years. It has revolutionized breast imaging, as the most highly sensitive imaging test for breast cancer. It is an extremely valuable tool in the detection of occult breast cancer for high-risk screening and in the assessment of extent of breast cancer. The sensitivity of MRI for detecting breast cancer is very high, in the order of 90% [1] and over 90–95% in women at high genetic risk for breast cancer [2, 3]. Its specificity is somewhat lower and ranges from 72% to 97% [1, 4, 5] depending on the population studied. Because of its lower specificity, histological proof of lesions detected on MRI is an essential requirement. Given the higher sensitivity of MRI compared with mammography and ultrasound, many lesions are only visible on MR and require MRI image guidance for proof of histology. Biopsy devices using MR-guidance and protocols for MRI-guided biopsy have been standardized [6, 7]. The ability of a center to offer MRI biopsy is very important, as it may offer lifesaving early diagnosis of breast cancer that might not otherwise be diagnosed (Fig. 5.1). This is increasingly relevant as the indications for breast MRI have expanded [8].

> **Key Point**
> MRI biopsy is an essential breast imaging technique that may provide a lifesaving early diagnosis of breast cancer in women in whom the cancer is not visualized by any other modality.

J. M. Seely (✉)
University of Ottawa, Ottawa, ON, Canada

Ottawa Hospital Research Institute, Ottawa, ON, Canada

The Ottawa Hospital, Ottawa, ON, Canada
e-mail: jeseely@toh.ca

© Springer Nature Switzerland AG 2019
C. M. Kuzmiak (ed.), *Interventional Breast Procedures*,
https://doi.org/10.1007/978-3-030-13402-0_5

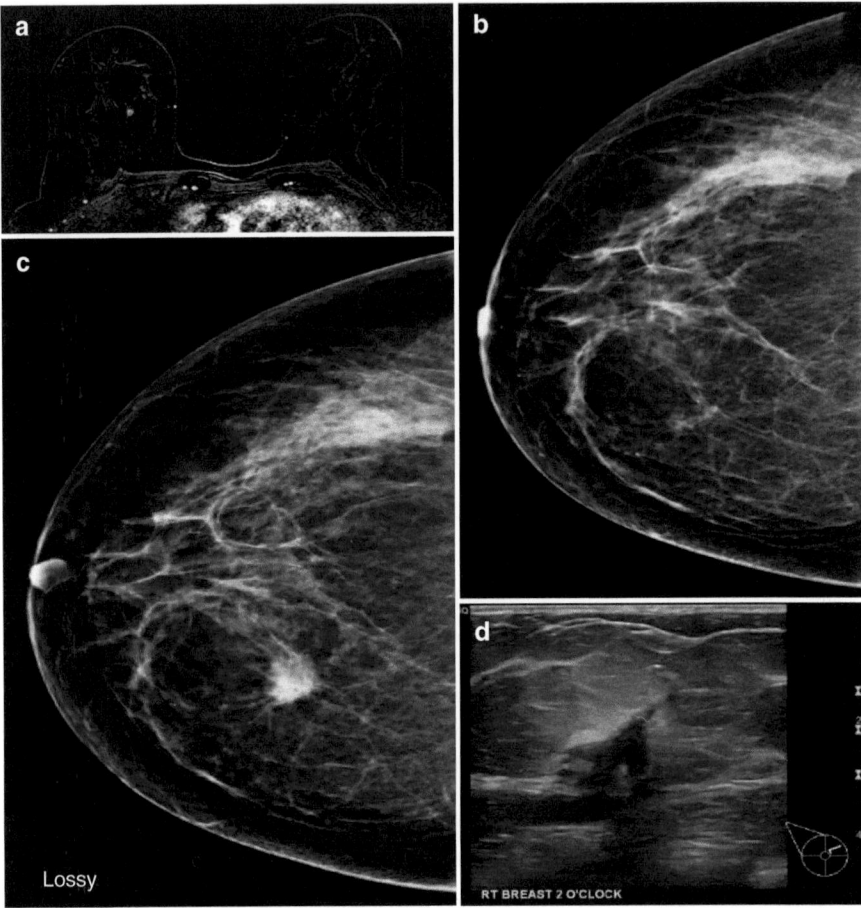

Fig. 5.1 A 52-year-old with 33% lifetime risk for breast cancer (IBIS). (**a**) Baseline high-risk screening MRI demonstrates a small rim-enhancing mass in the right breast on axial subtracted T1-weighted sequence 2 minutes post-gadolinium injection. (**b**) CC right mammogram view shows no corresponding mass. A second-look ultrasound at an outside institution (not shown) was reported as normal, and the patient was returned to annual screening. (**c**) Patient presented 11 months with a palpable mass at the same location. Diagnostic mammogram right CC view and (**d**) right breast ultrasound show interval development of a spiculated mass at same site as the MRI lesion. Final pathology was a 22 mm HER2+ ER+ grade 3, invasive ductal carcinoma ER+ PR+ and Her2 Neu positive with two axillary nodal metastases

Indications for Breast MRI

According to the American College of Radiology (ACR) guidelines, current indications for breast MRI include the following [8]:

1. Screening high-risk patients: Annual MRI is indicated for women with a lifetime risk of 20–25% or greater. This includes patients with known BRCA 1 or 2

mutations, as well as previous chest wall irradiation before the age of 30 and other risk factors. Several clinical trials have demonstrated the significant improvement in cancer detection that is otherwise mammographically and sonographically occult [2, 3, 9–14].

2. Screening intermediate-risk patients: Breast MRI may be considered as a supplement to mammography to screen women at a moderately elevated risk for breast cancer (15–20%), for example, and is recommended for women with a personal history of breast cancer and dense breast tissue or for those diagnosed with breast cancer under the age of 50 [15].

3. Screening women with newly diagnosed breast cancer may detect at least 3–5% of occult contralateral breast malignancy in patients with MRI [16–19].

4. Screening women with breast augmentation such as silicon or saline implants and/or free injections of silicone, paraffin, or polyacrylamide gel in whom mammography is difficult.

5. Assessing extent of disease: MRI may be useful to determine the extent of disease and presence of multifocality and multicentricity in patients with invasive carcinoma and ductal carcinoma in situ (DCIS). Breast MRI detects 16% of additional disease in these patients and changes to more extensive surgery in 6.5% [20].

6. Evaluating metastatic cancer of unknown origin but suspected to be breast in origin.

7. Characterization of lesions when other diagnostic imaging such as ultrasound and mammography (with or without tomosynthesis) and physical examination are inconclusive for the presence of breast cancer and biopsy cannot be performed [21–24].

Indications for Breast MRI Biopsy

According to the ACR guidelines, breast MRI biopsies are indicated for the following [7]:

1. Lesions only seen on breast MRI that do not have a definite correlate on mammography of ultrasound (US), which are suggestive or suspicious for malignancy (BI-RADS® 4 and BI-RADS® 5)

2. Repeat biopsy when the initial biopsy results are nondiagnostic or discordant with the imaging findings

Contraindications to Breast MRI Biopsy

1. The only absolute contraindication to MRI-guided breast biopsy is the inability to visualize the target breast lesion at the time of biopsy, once the contrast injection has been done. This may be due to resolution of the lesion, such with hor-

monally stimulated breast tissue, or due to restricted arterial flow to the breast from excessive compression. A 6-month follow-up MRI is recommended to ensure adequate follow-up of such lesions [25].

2. Patients on anticoagulation medication may proceed with MRI biopsy; reports demonstrate no significant increased bleeding risks in these patients [26, 27].
3. General MRI safety precautions should be observed [7, 28].
4. Patient should be able to maintain a prone position in the breast coil for 50–60 minutes and be able to fit within the magnet while in the coil.
5. Limitations to MRI biopsy also include challenging locations of the lesion, which limit the ability to target the lesion safely. For example, lesions close to the chest wall, breast implants, or the skin surface may prevent safe targeting for biopsy. In this case MRI-guided clip placement may be performed to enable surgical localization.

The History of MRI Breast Biopsy

The experience with MRI procedures began with MRI-guided localizations. The first report by Heywang-Kobrunner et al. in 1994 described a prototype breast coil for MRI-guided needle localization [29]. Two different techniques were reported, the freehand technique [30], which was associated with a high rate of wire displacement and performed in the supine position, and a dedicated stereotactic device performed in the prone position for MRI-guided localization [29]. Orel and colleagues reported in the same time on initial experience with MRI-guided localization and biopsies in the prone position [31]. In 1997, Christiane Kuhl and colleagues described their experience with a stereotactic device for MR imaging-guided wire placement and core biopsy, with the patient in the semi-prone position [32]. There were technical challenges documented with the core needle biopsy technique [33]. The technique soon evolved into vacuum-assisted biopsies with the first vacuum biopsies described in 1999 by Heywang-Kobrunner et al. [34] and in 2003 by Dr. Lieberman [35]. In the early 2000s, a lack of availability of MR-guided interventions for lesion localization and core biopsy was identified as the major reason for delayed adoption of MR imaging in clinical practice [36, 37] (Fig. 5.2). Improvements in MR-compatible needles combined with more commercially available MR-compatible breast biopsy devices allowed faster and safer biopsies that were fully integrated into clinical practice. Since 2010, and reiterated in 2017, the American College of Radiology stipulates that "facilities performing breast MRI must have the capacity to perform mammographic correlation, directed breast ultrasound, and MRI-guided intervention, or create a referral arrangement with a cooperating facility that could provide these services" [8]. Today, all facilities offering MRI should be able to perform MRI biopsies.

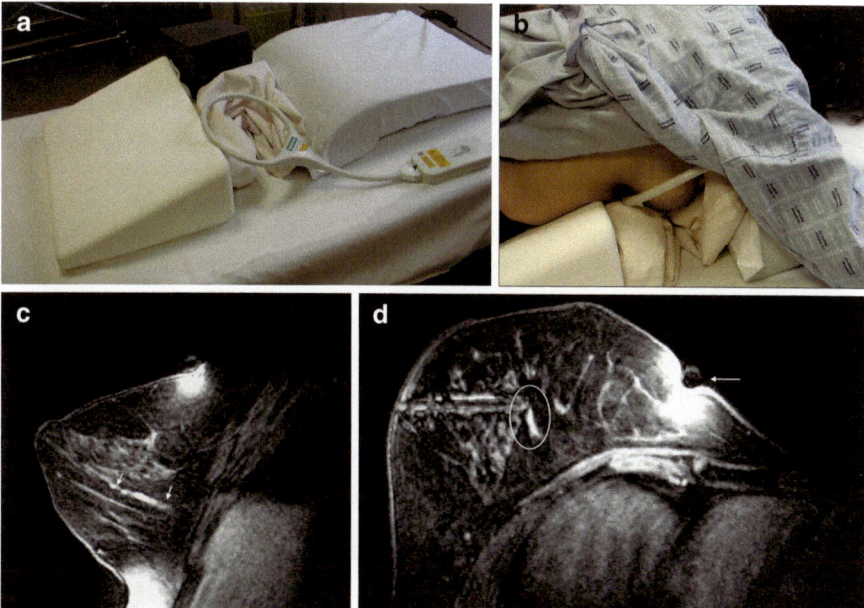

Fig. 5.2 Original setup in 2002 for MRI localization using a surface coil and freehand technique. (**a**) Setup with circular coil and support and breast mobilization with pads. (**b**) Patient lying prone in coil. (**c**) Sagittal T1 fat-suppressed image 5 minute post-contrast shows linear NME (arrows). (**d**) Localization needle (MR-compatible) targeting linear NME (circle). Note artifact from the circular coil (arrow)

Fundamentals

Breast MRI requires intravenous contrast to demonstrate vascularity of breast lesions. This may be related to tumoral neo-angiogenesis or to vascular benign lesions. Breast MRI lesions are described according to the ACR BI-RADS lexicon, and BI-RADS 4 or 5 lesions may present as an enhancing mass, a non-mass enhancement (NME) lesion, and/or a focus of enhancement (<5 mm) [38].

Basic Requirements of MRI Biopsy

Preparation

Second-Look Ultrasound

The first step in performing an MRI biopsy is to adequately prepare for the biopsy. This means reviewing the prior imaging, including the most recent mammograms and breast ultrasound. If a second-look ultrasound has not been performed for an

MRI lesion, this should be done prior to MR biopsy. A prior breast ultrasound that has not been targeted to the MRI finding is not sufficient.

The review is to ensure that a mammographic or sonographic correlate is not demonstrated, which would provide a more optimal target for biopsy. MRI breast biopsies are expensive and time-consuming, and ultrasound or stereotactic-guided breast biopsies are preferred methods of biopsy when possible. For any lesion detected on MRI, consideration to performing an MRI-directed ultrasound is recommended. If a suspicious MRI finding is identified with targeted ultrasound, then ultrasound-guided biopsy can be performed. Ultrasound-guided biopsy is the preferred method of biopsy as it is more comfortable for the patient, takes less time, and is less costly.

The frequency of an ultrasound correlate for MRI lesions varies between 23% and 82.1% [39–44]. A meta-analysis of 17 studies found a pooled rate of 57.5% [44]. The highest detection rates of second-look US are noted for mass lesions and malignant lesions [44]. Mass lesions identified on MRI are more likely to have a sonographic correlate than non-mass lesions (pooled estimates of 66% vs 29%) [44]. Larger enhancing masses and BI-RADS 5 lesions are more likely to be identified on second-look US with detection rates of 25–62% [39–43, 45]. Non-mass enhancement smaller than 1 cm and foci are less likely to be identified with second-look ultrasound, detected 11–42% [39–43, 45]. Given the low rate of US detection for non-mass enhancement <1 cm and foci, some centers proceed immediately to MRI biopsy.

The malignancy rate of MR-directed ultrasound-guided biopsies is reported from 4% to 56% with the pooled positive predictive value (PPV) of 30.7% [44]. Larger lesions are more likely to be malignant [46].

Experienced breast radiologists skilled at both MRI and US imaging modalities should only perform second-look US. Because the patient changes from prone in MRI to supine oblique position in US, the position of the lesion(s) must be carefully correlated to the quadrant location, depth in the breast and lesion to nipple distance, with correlation to landmarks such as fibroglandular tissue interface and adjacent cysts or masses. The change from prone to supine location commonly leads to lesion displacement and may occur over 3–6 cm, with the least movement occurring in the lesion to nipple and lesion to skin distances [47]. US correlates to MRI lesions often appear benign on US evaluation and should be treated with a high level of suspicion, if concerning on MRI [40] (Fig. 5.3).

Key Points
- A second-look ultrasound should be performed for most MRI lesions and is most accurate when using the lesion to nipple distance.
- A sonographic correlate may be found in 57.5% of lesions and is most likely with masses and malignant lesions.
- The positive predictive value of a MR-directed ultrasound-guided biopsy is 30.7%.

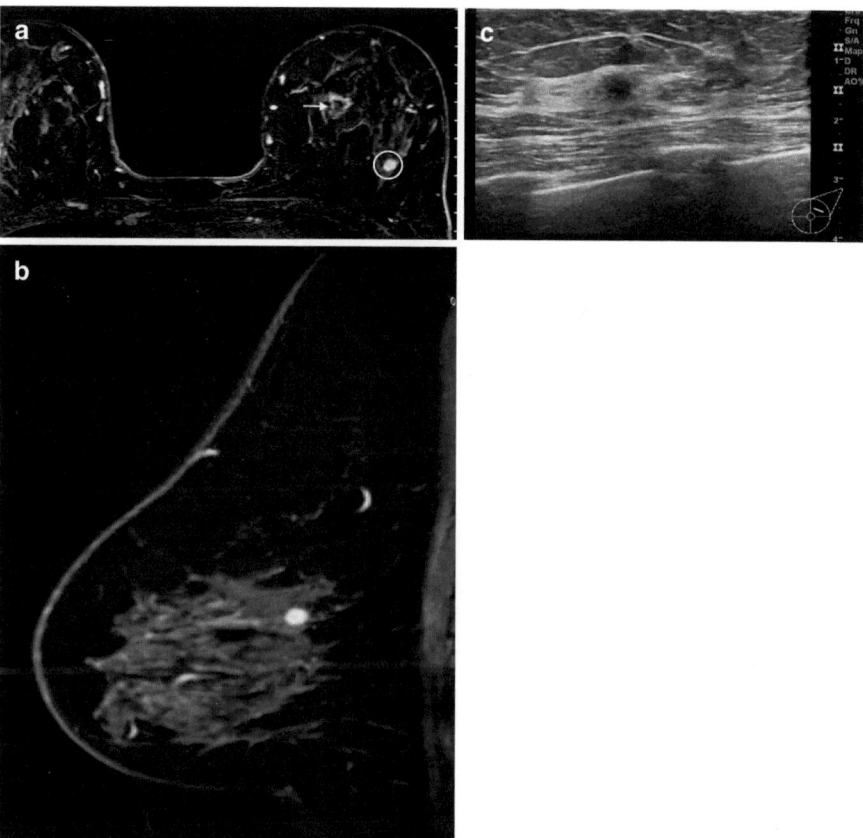

Fig. 5.3 Preoperative breast MRI done for extent of left DCIS disease. (**a**) Axial subtracted T1 image 2 minute post-contrast shows left DCIS biopsy cavity (arrow) and 6 mm enhancing mass (circle) with washout in upper outer quadrant of the left breast suspicious for multicentric, invasive disease. (**b**) Sagittal T1 fat-suppressed post-gadolinium image at 5 minute post-contrast shows rim-enhancing mass. (**c**) Second-look US shows a 6 mm poorly circumscribed mass corresponding to the enhancing lesion at same distance from the nipple as the MRI lesion. US-guided biopsy of the lesion confirmed an invasive ductal carcinoma, low nuclear grade

Second-Look Mammogram

Additionally, the mammogram should be reviewed. This can be considered analogous to a "second-look" mammogram. It has been shown that adding conventional imaging to non-mass enhancement lesion characterization at breast MR imaging improves the diagnostic performance of radiologists, and accuracy in particular improved if mammography is used [48]. The presence of calcifications on mammography may correlate with NME and provides a target for stereotactic biopsy in DCIS (Fig. 5.4). The malignancy rate is over 90% in cases of NME > 20 mm when accompanied by microcalcifications in the same area [48].

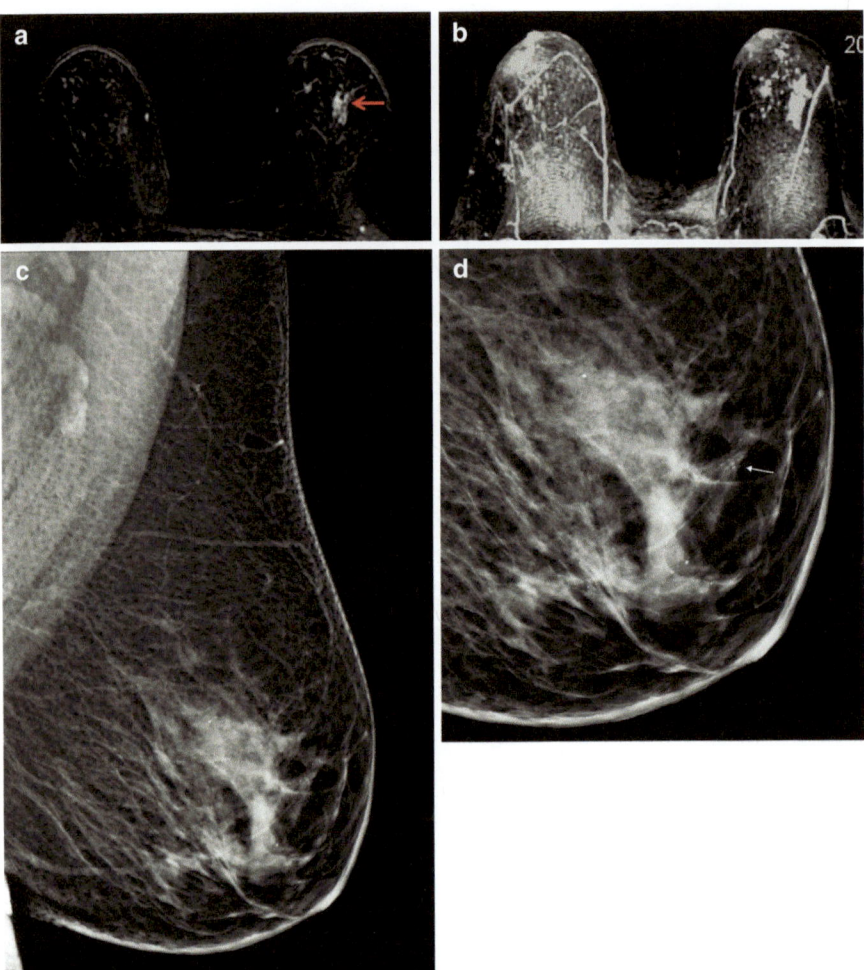

Fig. 5.4 A 65-year-old female with right biopsy-proven DCIS preoperative MRI. (**a**) Axial T1 subtracted image 2 minute post-contrast and (**b**) axial subtracted T1 MIP image show segmental NME in the upper outer quadrant of the left breast. The right DCIS biopsy site is not shown. (**c**) Second-look MLO left mammogram (initially reported as normal) and zoomed image (**d**) identify linear branching fine pleomorphic calcifications concerning for DCIS. Stereotactic biopsy confirmed high-grade DCIS

Second-Look Tomosynthesis

More recently, reports have shown that second-look digital breast tomosynthesis (DBT) may improve the detection of MRI findings. Clauser et al. found that second-look US found a correlate in 44/84 (52%), while digital mammography found 20/84 (24%) and DBT found 42/84 (50%), with the combination of second-look US plus DBT finding the most lesions: 63/84 (75%) (p < 0.001) [49]. In their study, the contribution of second-look DBT was most important for NME, where the increase in rate of findings went from 28% to 61% of lesions [49]. The improvement was noted for mass and NME lesions, size ≤ or > 10 mm, BI-RADS 4 or 5, and nonmalignant and/or malignant lesions. Another study of 520 patients evaluated preoperatively for extent of disease with MRI had 164 additional enhancing lesions. Of these, targeted US identified 114 (69.5%), while 50 (30.5%) were not identified, and DBT identified 32/50 (64%), increasing the overall characterization to 89% (146/164) [50]. Using DBT the identified lesions were significantly more likely to be malignant.

> **Key Points**
> - The combination of second-look US plus DBT finds the most MRI-detected lesions (75%).
> - The contribution of second-look DBT is most important for NME, with increase in rate of findings from 28% to 61% of lesions.

Clip Placement

For any biopsy site that appears to correlate with an MRI lesion, it is important to place a marker clip at the biopsy site. This allows confirmation that the correct location was biopsied and provides a target for subsequent surgical localization. Confirmation of the biopsy site is ideally performed with a post-procedure short MRI scan [5–53]. The MRI is performed with axial nonfat-suppressed T1-weighted sequences without contrast, in the breast coil, and takes less than 3 minutes to perform. The imaging relies on clip artifact and adjacent landmarks to demonstrate the correct biopsy location (Fig. 5.5). A study of 38 presumed US correlates underwent post-procedural MRI for clip verification and found 26% at a site distinct from the lesion originally identified on MRI, 10% of which ultimately revealed malignancy [54]. In another study by Meissnitzer and colleagues, follow-up imaging in 80 benign, concordant ultrasound-guided biopsies found the sonographic lesion did not correspond to the MRI finding in 10. Nine of these ten lesions underwent subsequent MRI-guided biopsy, and five cancers were diagnosed [45]. Therefore any suspicious lesion that was not correctly sampled on US-guided biopsy requires a repeat MRI-VAB biopsy. A useful rule of thumb is to avoid performing an US-guided breast biopsy unless the sonographic correlate to the MRI lesion is convincing to the radiologist.

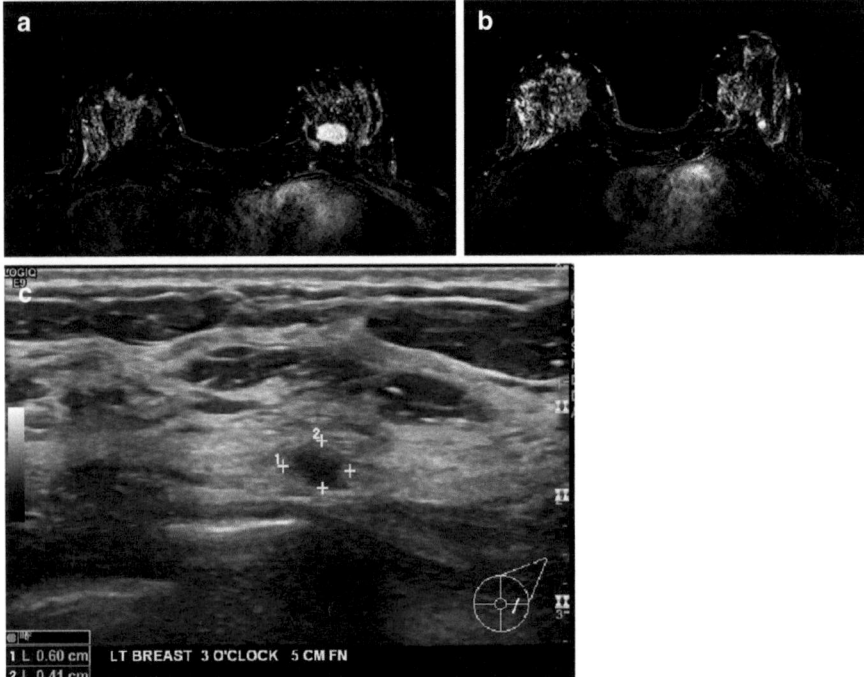

Fig. 5.5 A 50-year-old female with a 20 mm invasive ductal carcinoma at 7:00 in the left breast underwent preoperative MRI for extent of disease. Axial T1 post-gadolinium subtracted images (**a**) of enhancing mass at biopsy-proven cancer at 7:00 and (**b**) in lower outer quadrant, a second smaller enhancing mass concerning for a multicentric malignancy. (**c**) Second-look US found the presumed correlate. (**d**) MLO and (**e**) CC mammograms post-biopsy clip placement and (**f**) axial T1 nonfat-suppressed, non-enhanced image with signal void of clip artifact at biopsy site confirm accurate location of biopsy. Final pathology was a fibroadenoma, concordant with imaging findings. The lesion was not present on the follow-up MRI 6 months later in keeping with adequate sampling

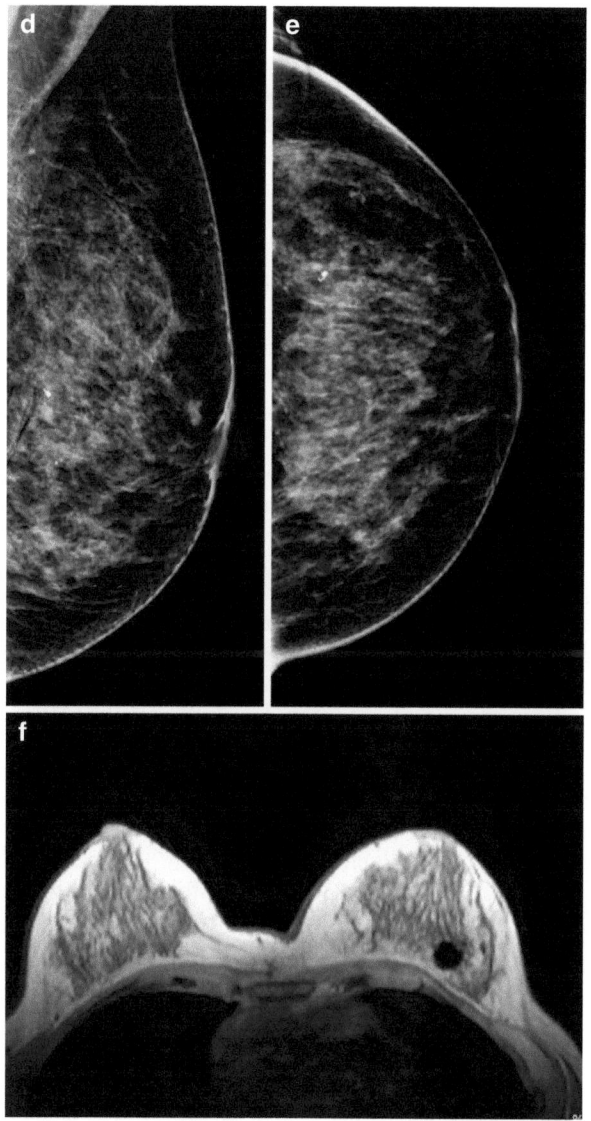

Fig. 5.5 (continued)

Rates of Malignancy in MRI Biopsies

The ACR BI-RADS lexicon recommends assigning a category BI-RADS 4 or 5 for a suspicious enhancing breast lesion on MRI before additional conventional imaging to allow helpful direction of management. If there is no correlate on conventional imaging of mammography, tomosynthesis, or second-look ultrasound, then the radiologist should recommend that an MRI breast biopsy be performed.

When a lesion is not visualized at second-look US, malignancy occurs in 12.2% of patients [44]. Therefore a negative second-look US does not exclude malignancy, and MRI biopsy is essential (Fig. 5.1). Rates of malignancy among series of MRI breast biopsies range from 20% to 50%, with a pooled rate from multiple studies of overall cancer yield of 36% [32, 33, 49, 55–63]. This depends on the population in which the MRI biopsies are being performed: in preoperative staging of extent of disease, the rate of positive MRI biopsies is reportedly much higher. In a preoperative evaluation of extent of disease, occult at second-look US and tomosynthesis, 81% (17/21) MRI lesions were malignant [49].

Key Point
- Lesions presenting with ipsilateral breast cancer, washout kinetics, and non-mass enhancement in the setting of preoperative evaluation have a higher PPV of cancer than lesions detected in the screening population.

The positive predictive value of MRI-guided biopsy is lower than ultrasound-guided biopsy of MRI-directed lesions. The frequency of malignancy is much higher in patients undergoing diagnostic MRI (28%) vs screening (10%) and in patients with ipsilateral breast cancer (45%) and in lesions with washout kinetics (33%) and is 34% in lesions with NME, representing DCIS in the majority of cases [61].

Performing an MRI Biopsy

MRI-guided biopsy is a unique application in MRI, and breast biopsies require expertise in interventional breast biopsy technique, as well as training in breast MRI. Although there are no specific ACR recommendations for numbers of MRI biopsies to be performed or supervised, the European MR breast biopsy consensus guidelines recommend that the performing radiologist would have sufficient competence with VAB (>50 procedures per year) and over 15 MRI-guided VAB procedures, maintaining experience with 10 or more MRI-VAB procedures per year [6]. In the UK, the National Health Service Breast Screening Programme (NHSBSP) guidelines recommend that experienced breast centers perform at least 12 MRI-guided breast biopsies per year and within centers that have recognized expertise in over 50 image-guided VAB procedures per year [64].

Consent

Consenting for the patient is an important part of the preparation for the biopsy. It establishes the communication between the radiologist and the patient and allows the patient to prepare for the biopsy. There is increasing evidence that women experience lower pain when the anticipated pain is less, which may be explained by the radiologist during the consenting process [65].

Positioning the Patient

The key to a successful MRI breast biopsy is proper positioning (Fig. 5.6). The breast must be deeply seated within the coil to facilitate access to posterior tissues (Fig. 5.7). Mammography technologists are familiar with this for prone stereotactic biopsy and are comfortable with this task. MRI technologists on the other hand have not been trained in this positioning and often require dedicated training to help with the positioning. It is very helpful for the radiologist to closely supervise the patient positioning and grid placement and to assist as needed. The radiologist should communicate to the technologist where the target is situated in the breast to ensure that the area is covered by the grid.

Patient positioning requires the patient to be comfortable during the procedure and maintain the same position for at least 40 minutes. Although padding may increase the comfort of the patient, it can reduce the depth of the breast within the coil. Therefore a balance is required between patient comfort and access.

The patients' arms should be considered during positioning. Patients may be more comfortable with their arms by their sides, but the coil and magnet size may limit this for large body habitus patients.

Contrast Enhancement

In pregnancy, gadolinium crosses the placental barrier and enters the fetal circulation, excreted through the fetal kidneys into the amniotic fluid. The potential bioeffects of gadolinium-based contrast agents are not well understood and recommended to be avoided [66]. Only a minuscule amount of gadolinium administered to a lactating woman is excreted into the breast milk and absorbed by the infant's gut; for this reason gadolinium-based contrast agents are considered safe, and cessation of nursing for 24 hours is considered unnecessary [66]. If there is concern on the part

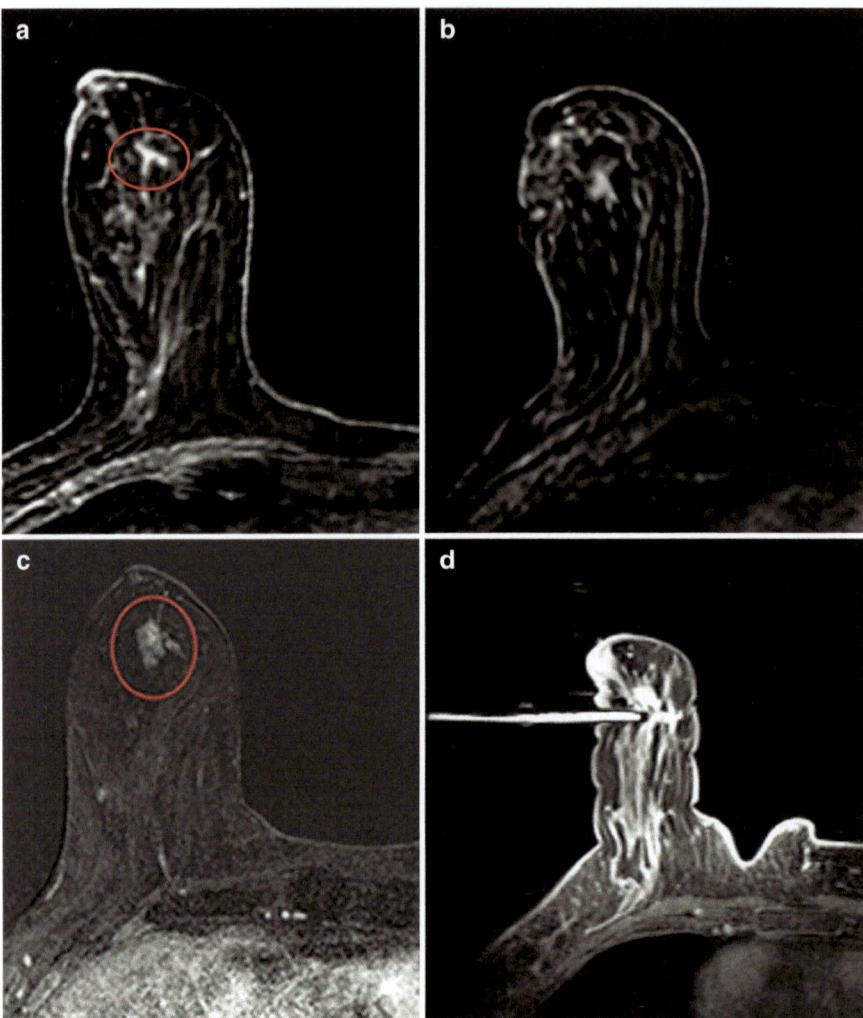

Fig. 5.6 High-risk screening MRI study. (**a**) Axial 2-minute post-contrast subtracted T1 image shows a new linear branching NME in the retroareolar right breast. A stereotactic biopsy was performed for coarse heterogeneous calcifications (not shown) in the same area, and results were fibrocystic changes, which were reported as concordant. (**b**) The patient returned only 14 months later for follow-up MRI that showed suboptimal positioning, and findings were reported as stable. (**c**) Screening MRI 13 months later showed interval growth of the retroareolar NME. (**d**) MRI biopsy provided a diagnosis of invasive lobular carcinoma grade 2/3 (pT1cN0) with LCIS treated by lumpectomy

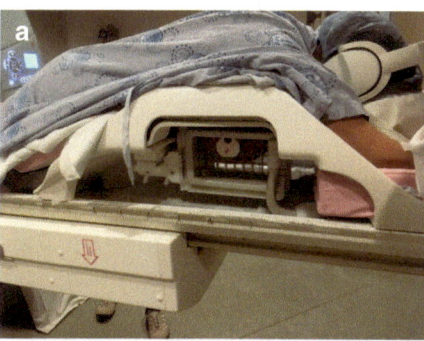
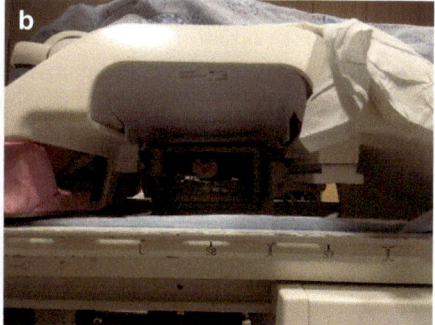
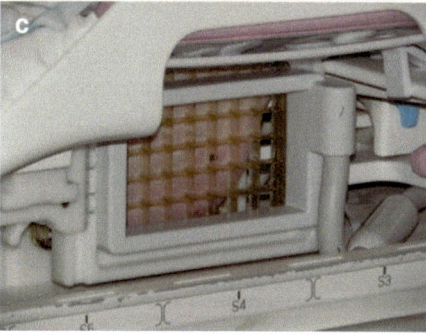

Fig. 5.7 Patient is positioned in the breast coil to allow for both (**a**) lateral and (**b**) medial approaches, with fiducials in place on lateral and medial grids. (**c**) Patient is positioned with the breast gently compressed in the grid, with a planned lateral approach. The lateral fiducial has been removed, and the site of the planned needle insertion has been marked on the skin

of the referring physician or patient, the nursing mother can be advised to discard her breast milk for 24 hours after GBCA administration.

Contrast should be injected at 0.1 mmol/kg with a 3 cc/sec flow rate and a 20 ml bolus of saline. The contrast arrival in tissue should coincide with the center of K-space (20 seconds from the start of the injection).

Technique

General Principles

- MRI biopsies require specific MR-compatible equipment.
- The breast tissue must be immobilized to allow needle entry.

- The patient must be supported in the prone or semi-prone position to allow access to the breast from a medial or lateral approach.
- Gentle compression is recommended between two compression plates.
- A grid must be placed within the compression plate and against the breast to allow for needle fixation and localization.
- An MR fiducial must be placed in the grid to allow lesion localization.
- The patient must be able to be moved in and out of the magnet to allow tissue sampling.
- Large bore vacuum-assisted biopsy needles are required for tissue sampling.
- Contrast injection is required to confirm the presence of the enhancing lesion.
- The lesion must be visible to allow insertion of the needle at the correct location.
- There should be visual confirmation of lesion sampling during the MRI biopsy.
- A follow-up breast MRI 6–12 months post-biopsy is required to confirm adequate sampling of the lesion.
- A clip must be placed at the biopsy site to allow identification of the lesion or biopsy site for surgical removal.
- A post-procedure mammogram should be performed to ensure correct location of the clip at the biopsy site.

Step-by-Step Approach to Performing an MRI Breast Biopsy

- The patient is first consented for the biopsy, with time for the patient to ask questions. The procedure should be explained to the patient, and she should consent to all parts of the biopsy, including the clip placement and mammogram required after the biopsy is completed. The patient is prepared with completed MR safety checklist and intravenous access, and the patient is double gowned to easy access of the breasts within the interventional breast coil. The patient is then brought into the MRI suite.
- The equipment consists of 8–12 G commercially available MRI-compatible vacuum-assisted biopsy device, including the introducer kit and needle. The 10G biopsy device is illustrated here (Fig. 5.8). Blunt tip needles (reduced dead space) are also available which may help for lesions close to the skin surface on the opposite side.
- The technologist assists in placing the patient prone in the breast coil. One or both breasts may be placed in the breast coil for imaging depending on whether a bilateral biopsy is being done. If a unilateral biopsy is performed, then the contralateral breast may be positioned close to the chest wall to allow access medially and laterally to the biopsy breast side (Fig. 5.7).
- The radiologist reviews the MRI images prior to positioning the patient and advises the technologist of the estimated site in the breast. For a posterior lesion close to the chest wall, the technologist may want to place the patient in a semi oblique prone position to allow more posterior breast tissue to be included in the grid. For very posterior lesions, positioning the patients' arms

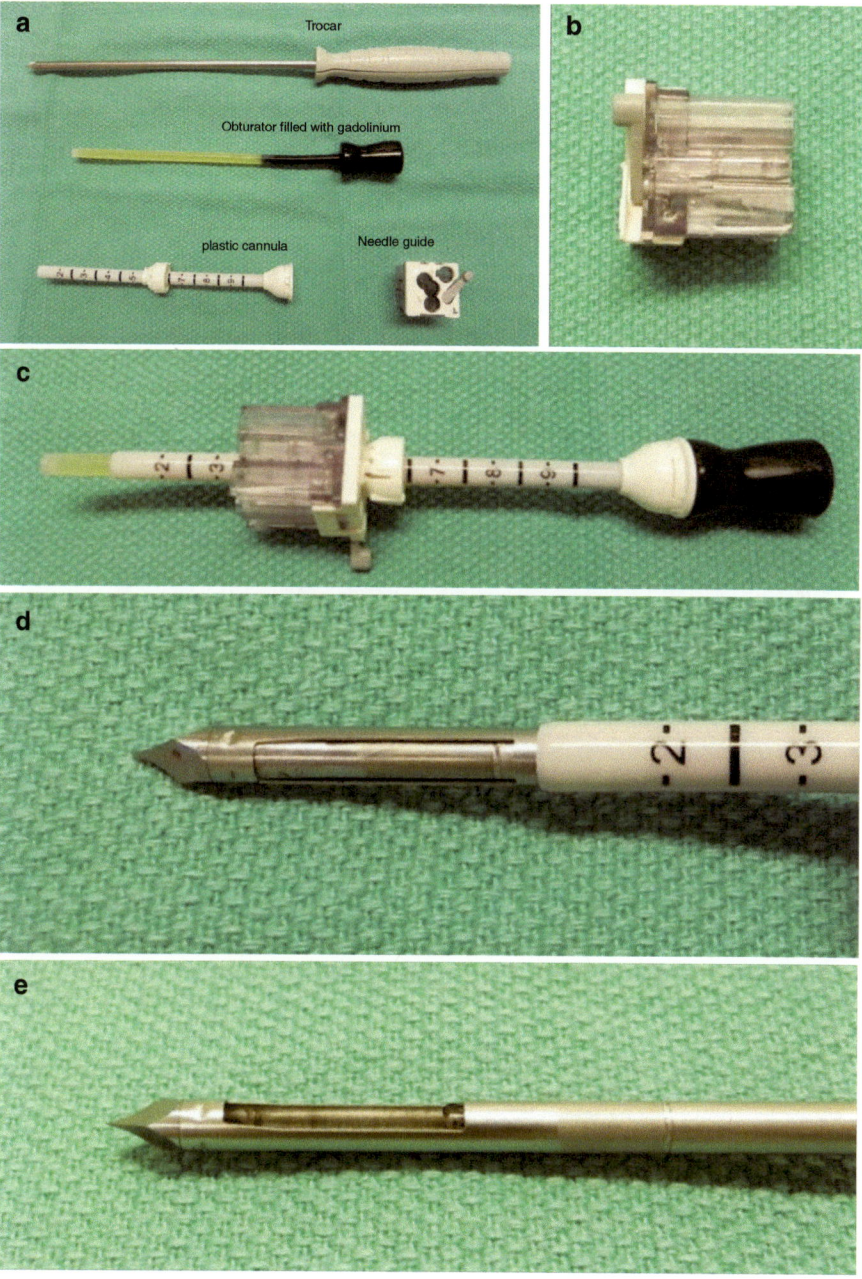

Fig. 5.8 Equipment for 10 G vacuum-assisted needle biopsy. (**a**) Image of trocar, obturator, plastic cannula, and needle guide block en face. (**b**) Needle guide block on side (2 cm thick). (**c**) Obturator in cannula and needle block. (**d**) Needle in cannula, center of sampling notch at 0. (**e**) Needle aperture open. (**f**) Picture of biopsy sampling through needle guide. (**g**) Picture of biopsy vacuum machine outside of the MRI suite. (**h**) Image of directional sampling ability with SenoRX device. (**i**) Collection chamber of vacuum needle filled with samples. (**j**) Diagram of distance of needle, dead space, and sampling notch

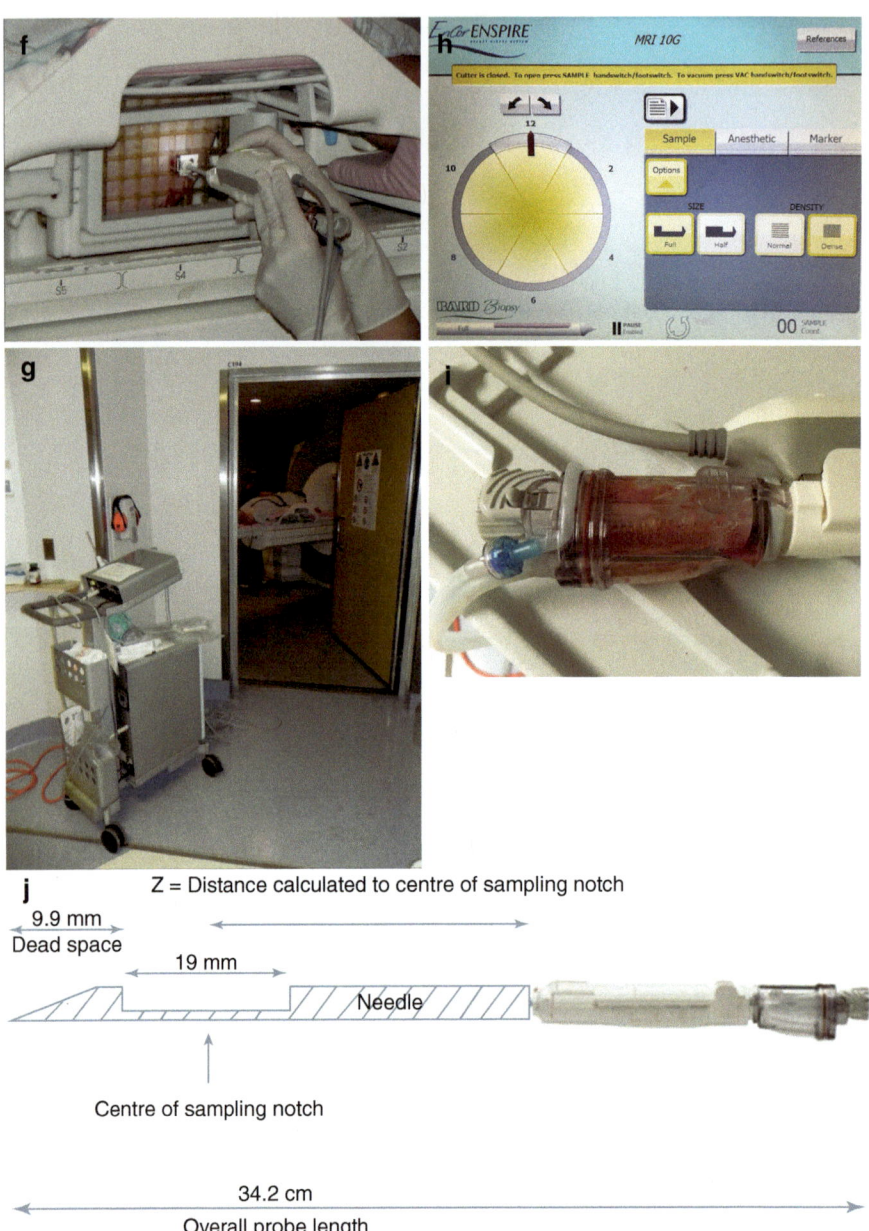

Fig. 5.8 (continued)

close to her side instead of above the head may allow for more posterior tissue to be included in the field.

- The breasts should be compressed gently between the compression plates. This means the tissue should be firmly in position but not taut, as excessive compression will lead to reduced blood flow to the breast tissue and may artificially prevent a lesion from enhancing. The nipple(s) should be positioned pointing to the bottom of the coil, and there should be no skinfolds or parts of the breast excluded from the coil. The patient should be comfortable and able to remain in this position for about 40–60 minutes.
- Once positioned, the technologist performs axial, sagittal, and coronal localizer sequences with the breast coil. The images of these sequences should be verified to confirm satisfactory positioning.
- Next axial and sagittal T1 pre-gadolinium sequences are obtained in the breast. The ideal is that they be obtained using fat suppression, although this is not essential so long as subtraction can be performed. The image slice thickness should be a maximum of 3 mm or less within plane pixel resolution of 1 mm or less [8]. The time to acquire the images should be a maximum of 4 minutes post-contrast injection [7]. Our practice is to obtain 1 mm thick slices through the breast in a 1-minute temporal resolution. These images are verified by the radiologist for satisfactory position of the expected location of the lesion and the grid. If there are concerns about the coverage of the grid over the expected location of the lesion, the patient may be repositioned before starting the study.
- Once the correct position is confirmed and the pre-gadolinium images are satisfactory, the contrast using gadolinium is injected intravenously. Scanning may begin as early as 1 minute post-contrast injection and no more than 4 minutes after contrast injection. This will ensure that rapidly enhancing lesions, which are more often malignant, are better demonstrated than more slowly enhancing benign lesions or fibroglandular tissue. The images are sent to the biopsy software program, if available, and images are reviewed using subtraction to confirm that the lesion is present. If the lesion is not present, a second series of images may be obtained, 4–6 minutes postinjection (Fig. 5.9). This may confirm that more slowly enhancing lesions, particularly non-mass enhancing lesions, are visualized. If the lesion is confirmed to be present, then the coordinates to target the lesion are obtained from the software program or using a manual calculation (Figs. 5.10 and 5.11). A general rule of thumb is to select the shortest distance to the target, except for cases that may be too close to the skin or for posterior lesions that may require a lateral approach.
- The depth of the lesion, the location relative to the fiducial on the grid, and the location of the needle within the grid plug are the three essential data points required to perform the breast biopsy. Once the targeting is calculated, the infor-

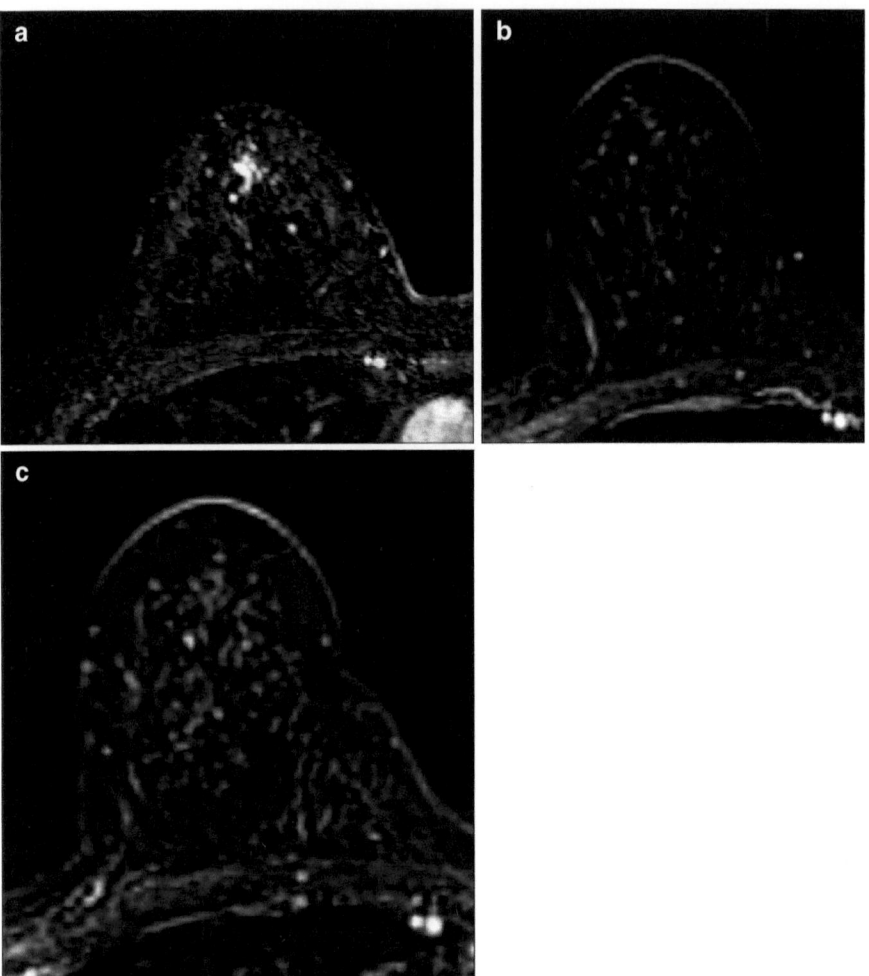

Fig. 5.9 (**a**) High-risk screening MRI shows a clumped area of NME in the right superior breast at 12:00 on axial T1 subtracted contrast-enhanced MRI at 2 minutes post-contrast. (**b**) On the day of MRI biopsy, there was no enhancement of the right breast lesion at 2 minutes and (**c**) 6 minutes post-contrast. The biopsy was cancelled and a 6 month follow-up MRI (not shown) was normal. The enhancing area was consistent with hormonally stimulated breast tissue

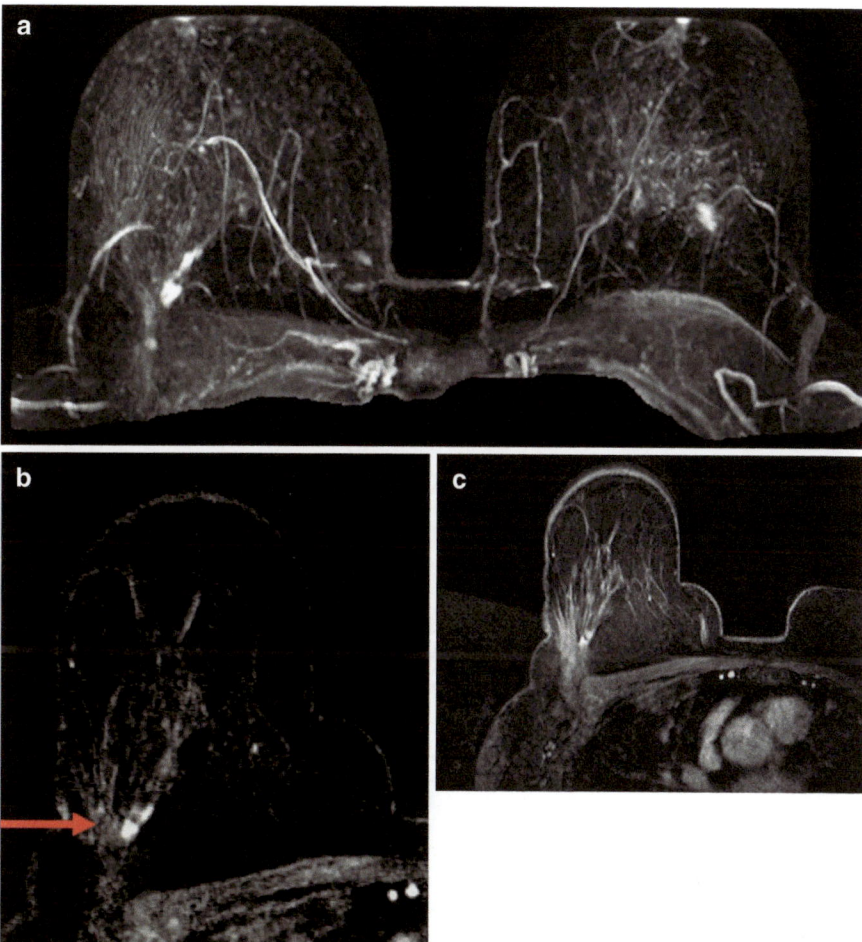

Fig. 5.10 Manual targeting in a woman with previous right breast cancer and confirmed recurrent carcinoma with MRI biopsy. (**a**) MIP of breasts demonstrates suspicious mass and NME in right breast upper outer quadrant. (**b**) On the day of the biopsy, the axial subtracted contrast-enhanced T1 sequence before placing needle demonstrates the persistent enhancing mass in the right breast (arrow). (**c**) Post-gad non-subtracted T1-weighted image of mass (**d**) measuring the distance from the skin to the lesion in breast (23 mm). *2 cm for the thickness of the plug must be added to the calculation of the depth.* (**e**) Sagittal fat-suppressed non-subtracted image of lesion. (**f**) Sagittal image of coil with Vitamin E capsule (arrow). By scrolling to the site of the lesion on the sagittal images, the radiologist could mark the site on the grid (circle) for needle placement. (**g**) Axial T1 fat-suppressed image confirms accurate location of the needle at the mass (not visible due to increased contrast enhancement of the adjacent scar tissue, in keeping with "vanishing target"). (**h**) Post-biopsy axial and sagittal. (**i**) T1 fat-suppressed sequences confirm signal void at biopsy site. (**j**) Close-up view of post-biopsy MLO shows biopsy cavity adjacent to surgical clip from previous lumpectomy and new "M" clip from MRI biopsy site

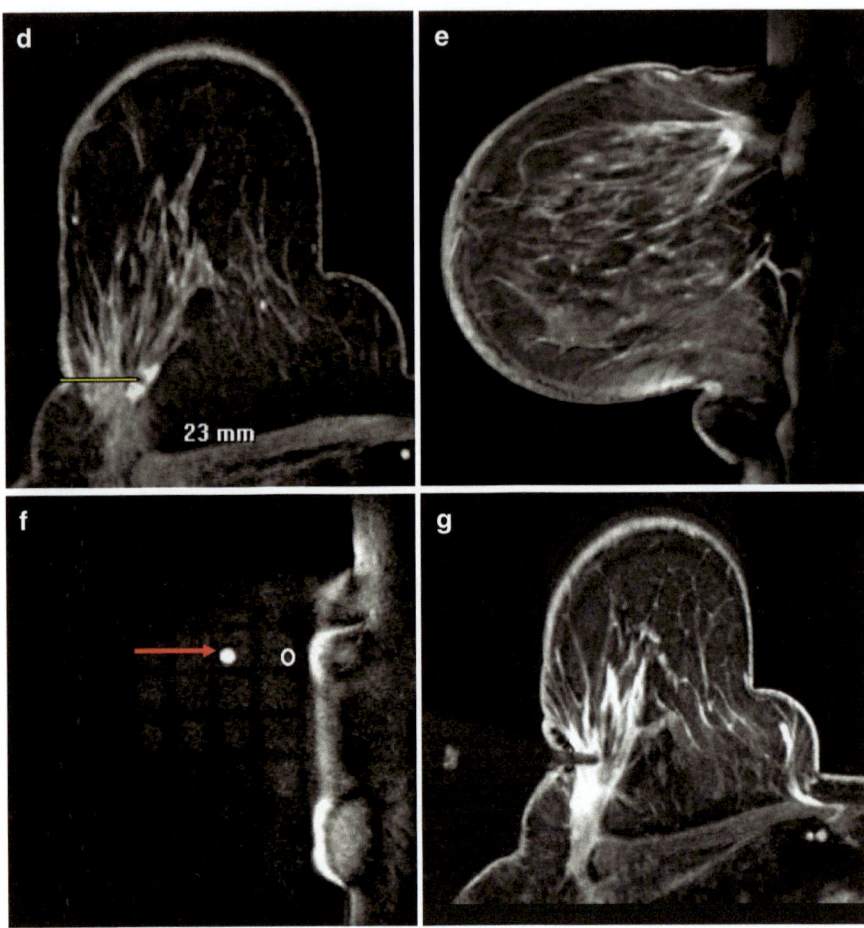

Fig. 5.10 (continued)

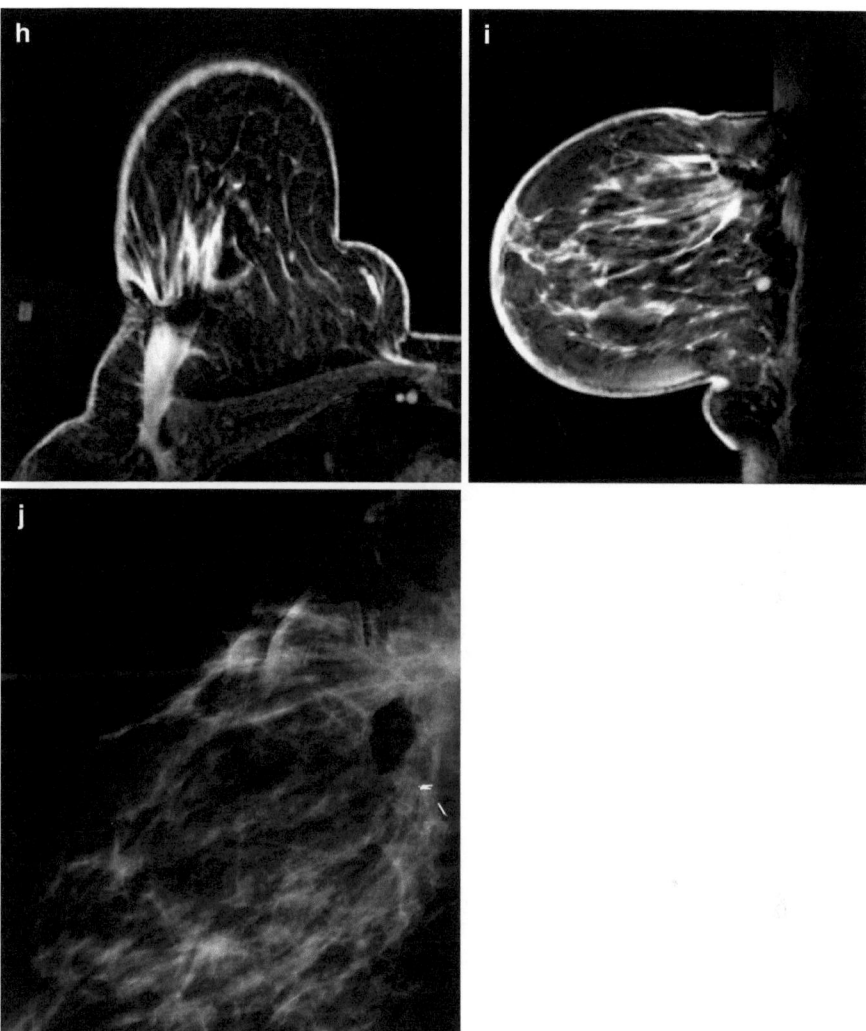

Fig. 5.10 (continued)

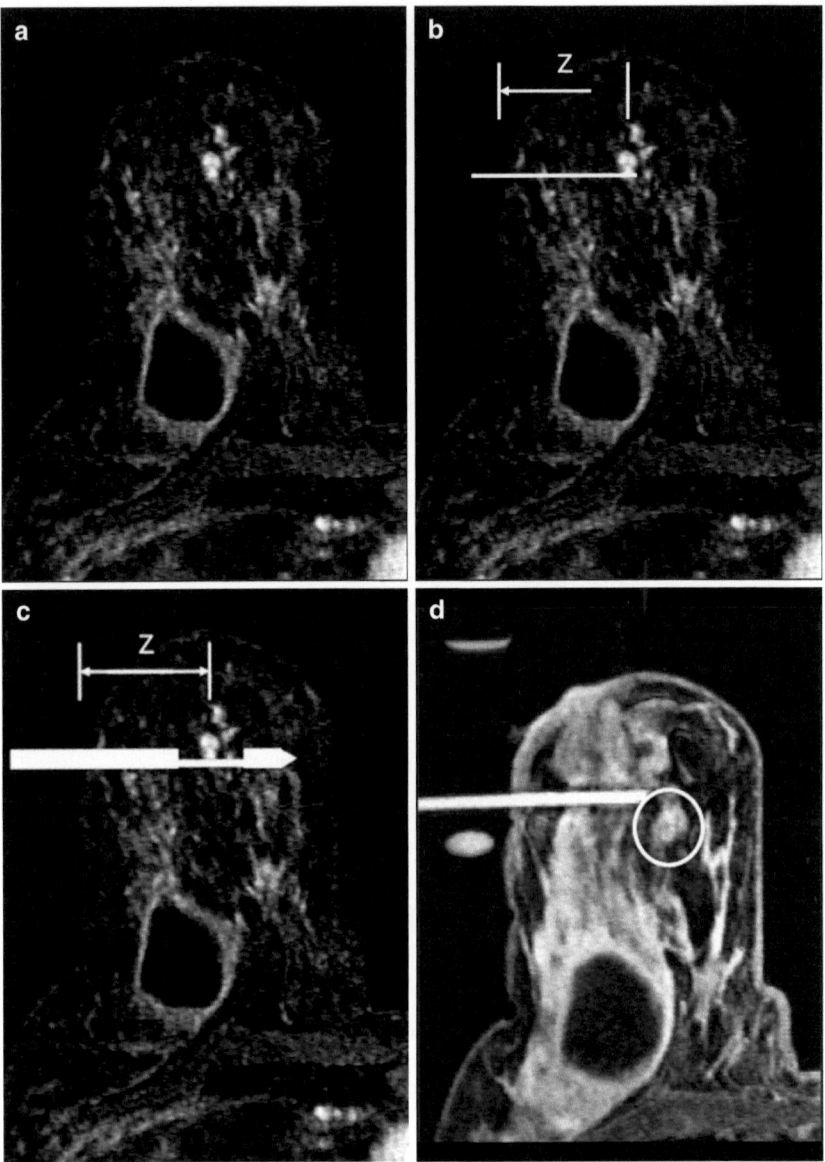

Fig. 5.11 Manual targeting in a woman at high risk for breast cancer with mass on screening MRI and no US correlate. (**a**) Axial subtracted contrast-enhanced T1 sequence before placing needle demonstrates the persistent enhancing mass in the right breast. (**b**) Manual calculation of distance from surface plug to the center of the mass, adding 2 cm for the needle plug thickness. (**c**) Estimated sampling notch with the mass at the center. (**d**) Axial and (**e**) sagittal T1 fat-suppressed images post-needle insertion confirm location of the needle with the mass (circle) displaced slightly posterior and superior to the obturator (arrow). (**f**) Axial and (**g**) sagittal post-biopsy T1 sequences show signal void at biopsy site; directional sampling of the mass superiorly and posteriorly enabled accurate sampling. (**h**) MLO and (**i**) CC post-procedure biopsy mammograms show biopsy clip within the biopsy cavity, in good position. (**j**) MLO and (**k**) CC right mammograms obtained following hook wire localization of biopsy-proven carcinoma. (**l**) Lumpectomy specimen radiograph confirming resection of biopsy clip, mass and wire

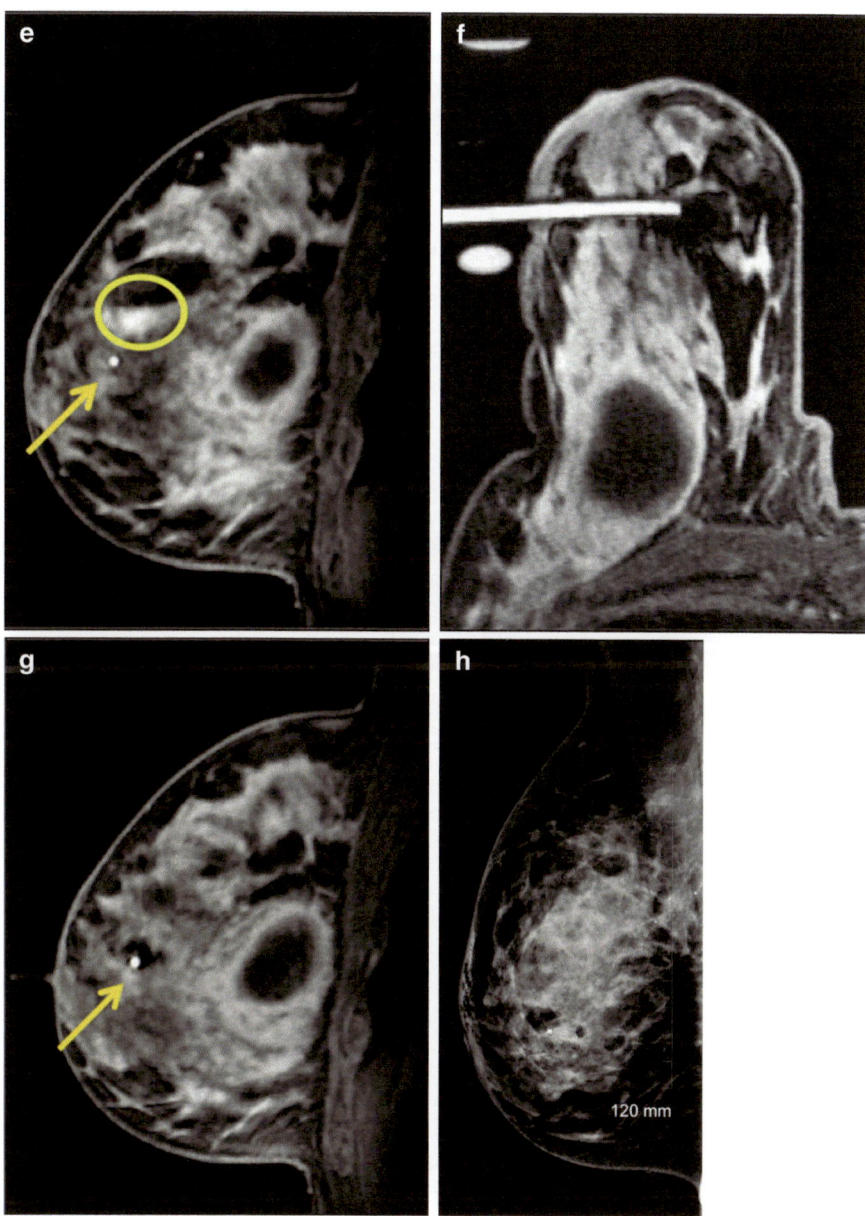

Fig. 5.11 (continued)

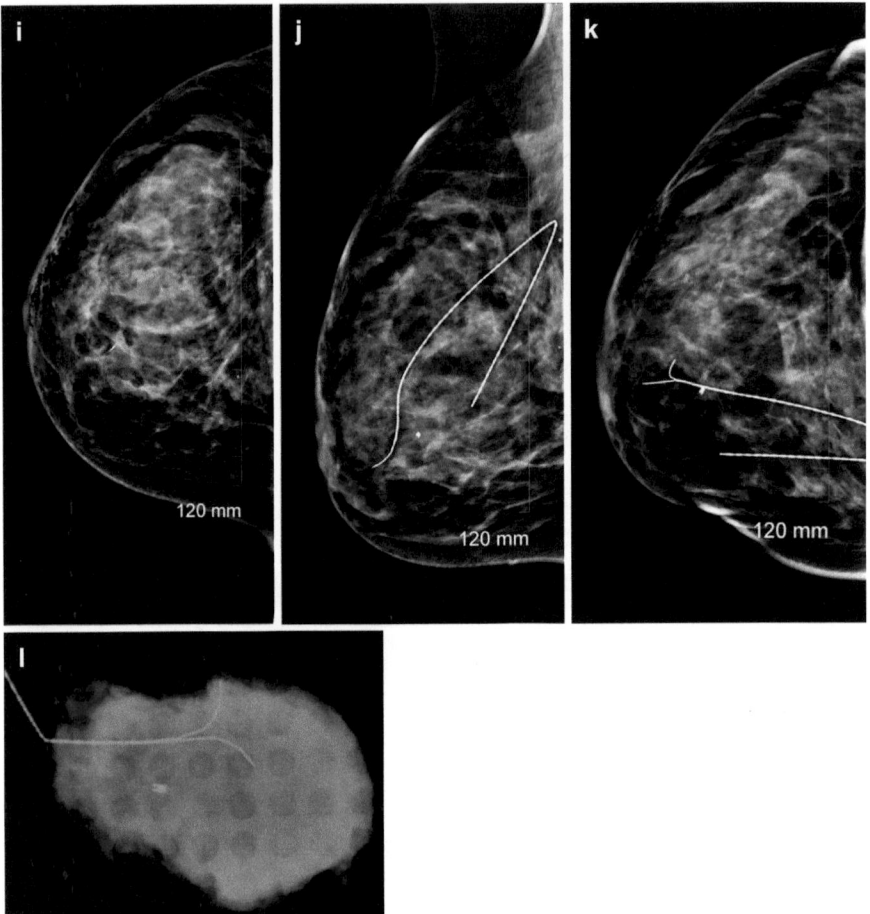

Fig. 5.11 (continued)

mation is written or printed on a paper that is brought into the MRI suite for reference by the radiologist (Fig. 5.12).

- In the MRI suite, the patient is slid out from the magnet, on the table taking care not to lose the patient's position on the MRI console. The patient is notified that the biopsy will proceed. The skin is marked at the site of the correct location for needle insertion. The skin is sterilized (cleansed) with alcohol or iodine-containing cleanser, and the local anesthetic is introduced (Fig. 5.13).
- Once satisfactory anesthetic is in place, a small incision is made in the skin with a scalpel, the incision parallel to the chest wall for optimal cosmesis. Then the plastic cannula and trocar are introduced into the breast through the grid plug. Tenting of the skin should be avoided (Fig. 5.14). The correct depth is confirmed, and the cannula is locked into position in the plug by rotating it clockwise. The trocar is then removed from the plastic cannula taking care not to change its

depth, and the obturator is inserted into the cannula. Once in place, the patient is placed back into the scanner for repeat imaging.

- Multiple or bilateral sites may be performed before repeat imaging (Fig. 5.14).
- Repeat imaging consists of the same axial and sagittal T1 sequences as used before. The images should be checked for accuracy of the obturator position, where the tip of the obturator should be at or within the lesion. The depth of the obturator is calculated to be central within the sampling notch of the biopsy needle, and biopsy cavity will therefore occur around this site. If the tip of the

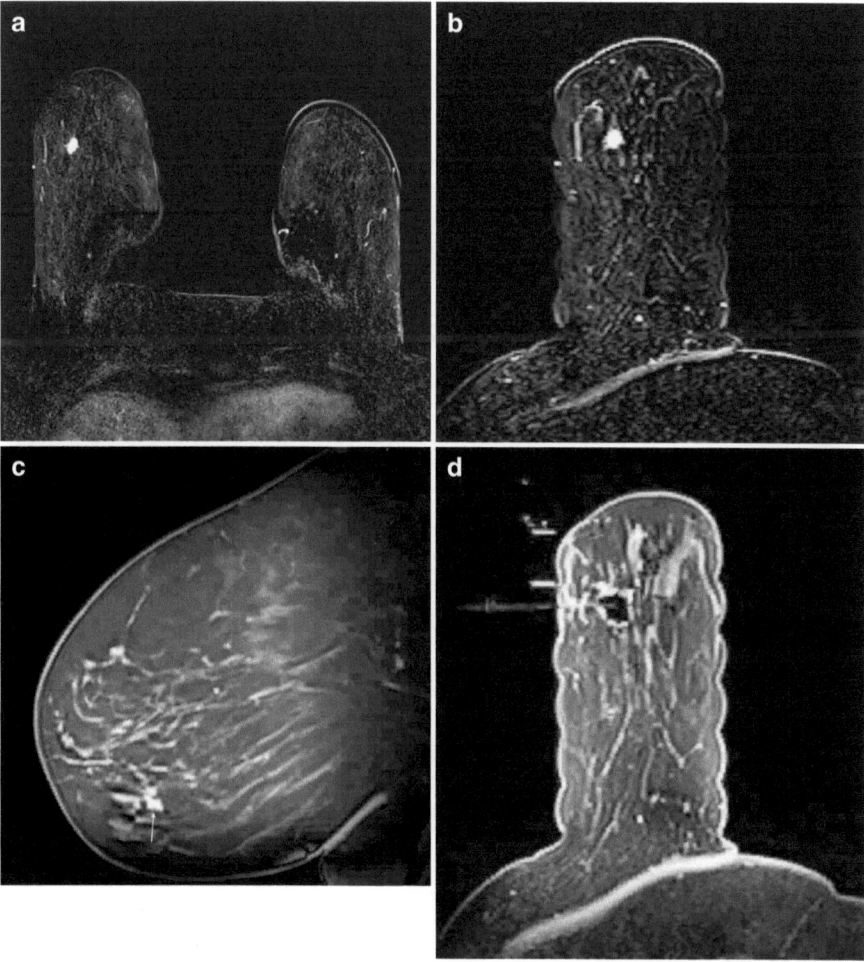

Fig. 5.12 High-risk screening MRI. (**a**) Axial subtracted T1-weighted sequence shows an irregular mass in the lower outer quadrant of the right breast that had increased since the previous year. (**b**) Axial subtracted and (**c**) sagittal fat-suppressed post-contrast images of the mass (arrow) confirm it is present; (**d**) post-biopsy image shows resolution of the mass on axial image, and (**e**) sagittal image shows signal void at biopsy site with no residual mass

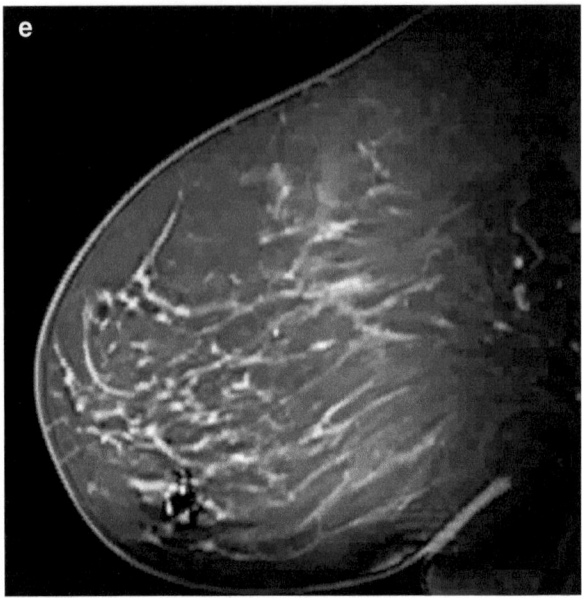

Fig. 5.12 (continued)

obturator is not adjacent to the lesion, and may have pushed the lesion away along the z-axis, as frequently occurs [67], then the trocar or needle may be used to advance the cannula to the correct depth. Likewise, repositioning of the needle with respect to location should be performed as needed and may be necessary if the patient moved or there were errors in the calculations. If repositioning is required, a repeat scan with axial and sagittal sequences may be required for confirmation of correct position.

- Once the cannula is confirmed in satisfactory position on axial and sagittal images, then the obturator is removed, and the biopsy needle is introduced into the cannula. Biopsy sampling may begin with verification that satisfactory anesthesia is in place. If the patient experiences any pain, more anesthetic should be inserted into the biopsy site, preferably through the needle itself but can be done through the cannula using a separate needle. At least 6–12 samples are obtained with the vacuum-assisted biopsy needle. Once the samples have been obtained, the needle is removed and the obturator is placed into the cannula. The specimens are fixed in neutral buffered formalin (4%) [6].
- The patient is again scanned in the MRI using the same axial and sagittal sequences. The images are verified to confirm that the lesion has been adequately sampled. If the radiologist notes insufficient sampling, then additional samples of the correct site using directional sampling should be obtained.
- Once sufficient sampling is confirmed, then the obturator is again removed, and a clip marker is deposited at the biopsy site, through the cannula, ensuring it is at the correct depth. Because the biopsy cavity is filled with air, blood, and contrast,

Fig. 5.13 Steps for needle biopsy. (**a**) Insertion of local anesthetic at correct site in the grid. (**b**) Scalpel incision for needle insertion site. (**c**) Insertion of needle guide with trocar and plastic cannula into correct position. (**d**) Trocar has been removed and obturator has been placed into the cannula. (**e**) Removing the breast coil from the compression plate and grid to allow access if necessary. (**f**) The obturator is removed, the 10G needle is introduced into the plastic cannula. (**g**) The needle is in good position within the cannula and is ready for sampling. (**h**) Image of the paper sheet on which are written or printed measurements for the depth of the introducer, the position in the needle plug, and the position on the grid, relative to the fiducial

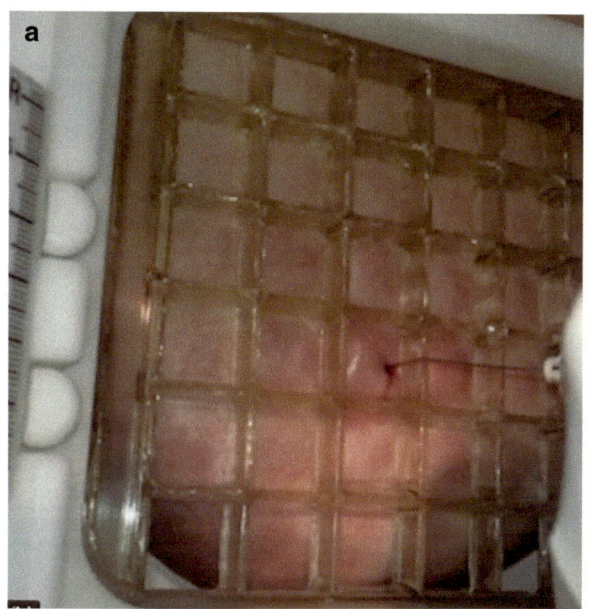

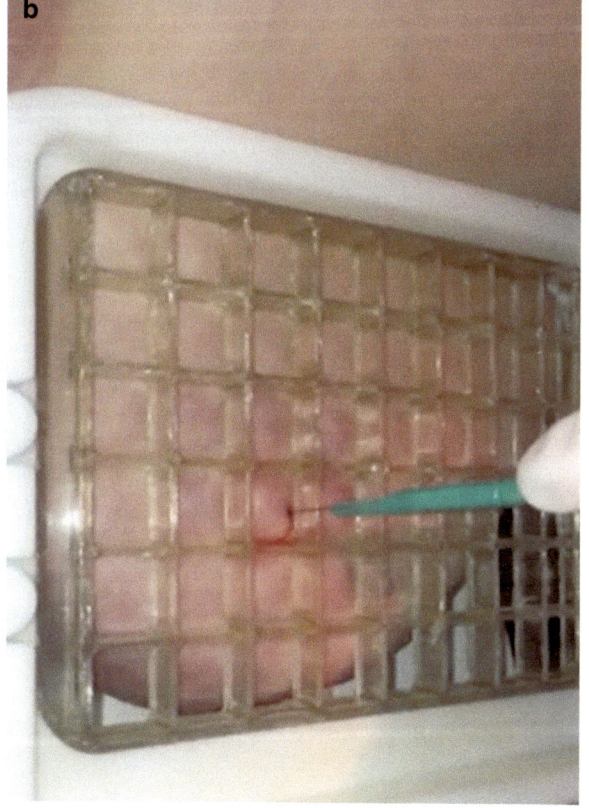

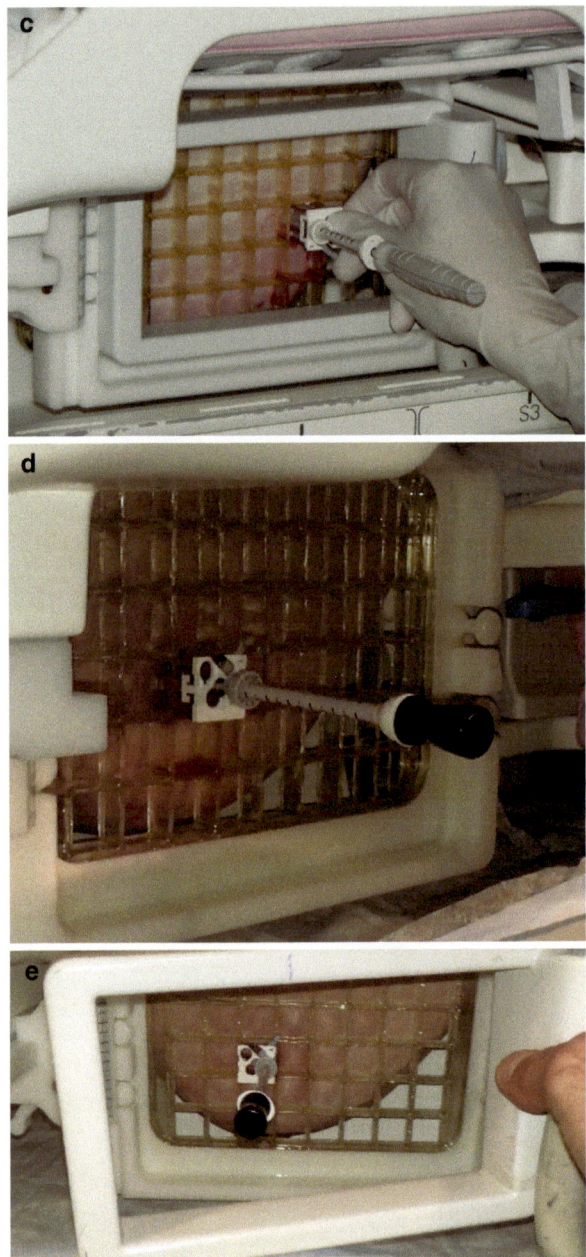

Fig. 5.13 (continued)

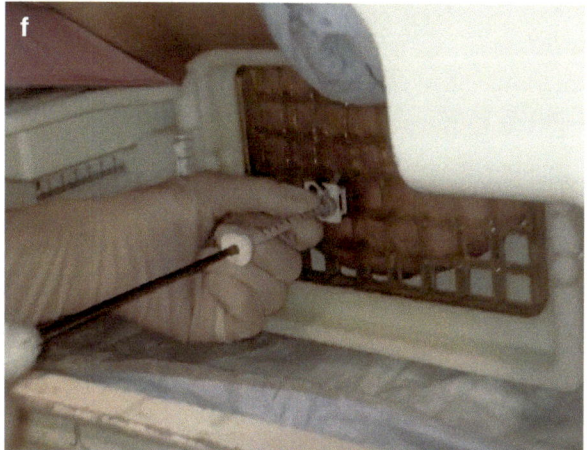

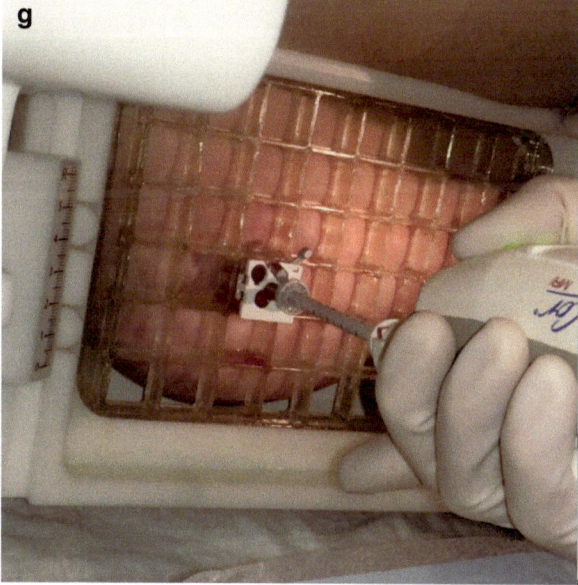

Fig. 5.13 (continued)

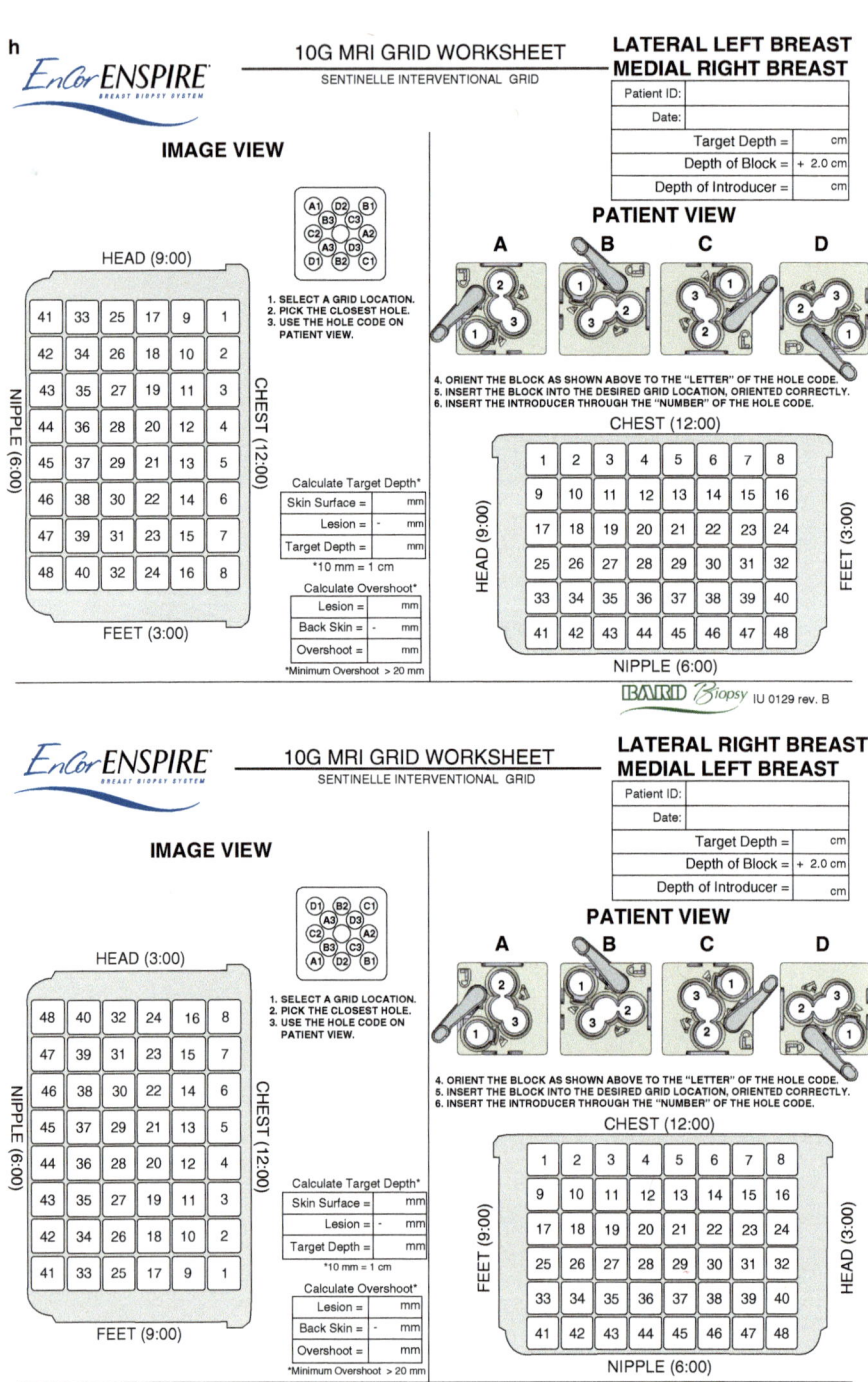

Fig. 5.13 (continued)

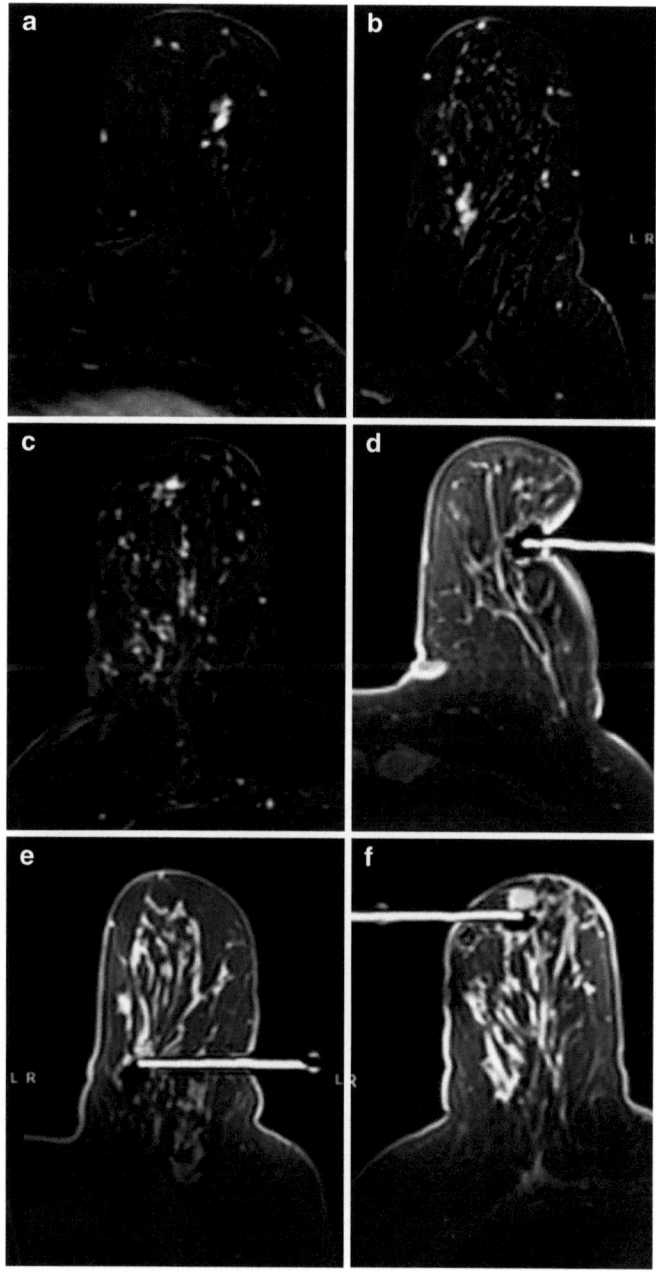

Fig. 5.14 High-risk screening MRI with multifocal NME and contralateral right focus, proven at MRI biopsy to be right LCIS and left sclerosing adenosis at both sites. (**a**) Axial subtracted T1 post-contrast image at 2 minutes shows linear NME in lower outer quadrant of left breast, (**b**) a separate NME in the left upper medial quadrant, and (**c**) contralateral right retroareolar focus. (**d**) Post-MRI biopsy imaging of left LOQ shows tenting of the skin at the entry, (**e**) left UMQ, and (**f**) right retroareolar sites

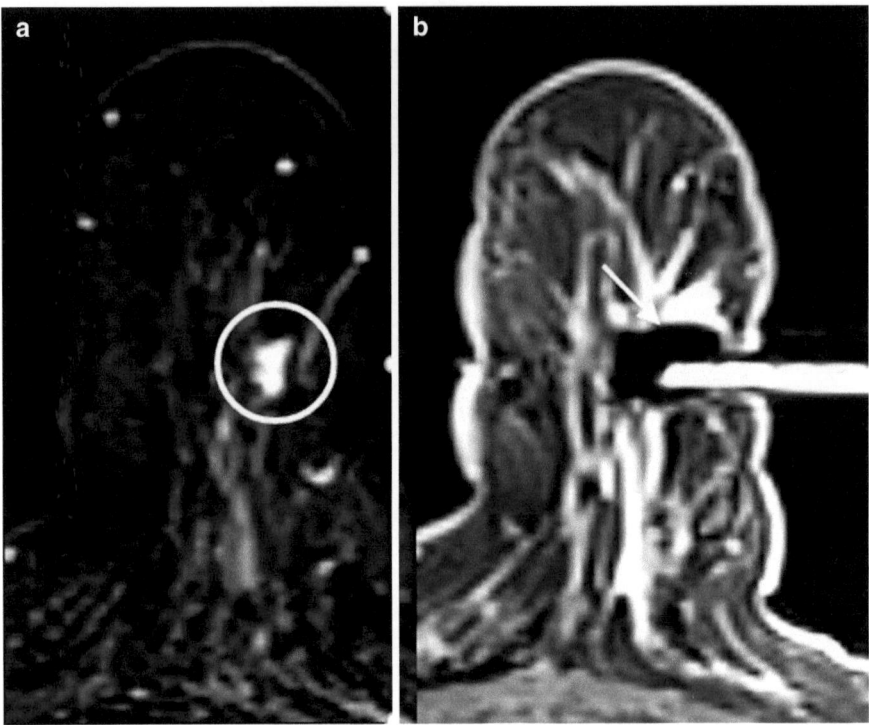

Fig. 5.15 (**a**) Subtracted axial image 2 minute post-gadolinium enhancement demonstrates a small irregular 7 mm mass in the breast. (**b**) Post-biopsy axial image with introducer in place and signal void at site of biopsy cavity filled with air and blood. Small air-fluid level (arrow) within cavity is noted. The lesion is obscured but landmarks suggest adequate sampling. Final pathology confirmed a small invasive ductal carcinoma

there is no ability to visualize the clip, and imaging with MRI is not helpful to confirm the correct clip location (Fig. 5.15).

- The patient is then removed from the MRI and taken out of the breast coil, taking care to compress the breast at the biopsy site. The patient is taken to a stretcher or bed where she may recline and where manual compression is used to stop any bleeding. Generally, 5–10 minutes is sufficient to stop any bleeding and may help to reduce the formation of hematomas. The patient is bandaged and then directed to undergo a mammogram in CC and MLO views to demonstrate the correct location of the marker at the biopsy site.
- The radiologist will check the position of the clip before the patient leaves. In case of significant clip migration, i.e., more than 2 cm from the biopsy site, a second clip may be placed under ultrasound guidance using the biopsy hematoma as a landmark. Post-biopsy instructions are provided to the patient.
- An addendum report is added to the MRI biopsy report once the pathology results are received to confirm radiological-pathological concordance.

> **Key Points**
> - A clip should be placed at each MRI biopsy site.
> - If more than one lesion is being biopsied, a separate probe should be used for each to avoid cross contamination.
> - Following biopsy, a minimum of one post-biopsy MR sequence should be obtained to demonstrate the biopsy site and its relation to the targeted lesion.
> - Repeat sampling should be obtained if inadequate sampling has been obtained.
> - Post-procedure two-view mammograms should be obtained post-MRI biopsy to confirm accurate location of the clip at the biopsy site.

MRI-Guided Localization

For women in whom an MRI-guided biopsy is not possible, MRI-guided needle localization is an option to allow surgical excision of a suspicious breast lesion. For those lesions not amenable to MRI biopsy, solutions have included follow-up MRI (with the potential to delay diagnosis) or MRI-guided clip placement followed by mammographically guided needle localization and surgical excision, which may be subject to issues related to clip migration [68]. For this reason, MRI-guided localization is an attractive alternative.

Indications for MRI-guided localization [7]:

1. To guide excision of malignant lesions seen only on MRI or with discordant or nondiagnostic findings on MRI-guided core biopsy.
2. For lesions not amenable to MRI biopsy due to their location in the breast.
3. To allow complete excision of an MRI-demonstrated malignancy or high-risk lesion underestimated in size on mammography and/or ultrasound; MRI bracketing may be required.

Technique

An MRI-compatible 18-gauge needle and hook wire are inserted via a needle guide to the targeted depth with the tip of the needle located 2 cm beyond the target lesion. Additional sagittal and axial contrast-enhanced images are acquired to confirm satisfactory needle location, followed by wire deployment. Post-procedure two-view mammography is performed to show the wire position. In a study of 99 MRI-guided localizations, typical sites performed for needle localization were breast lesions in the subareolar, far posterior, or superficial (defined as <2 cm from the skin) aspect of the breast [68]. They found 38/99 (38.4%) cancers, 31 (31.3%) high-risk lesions, and 30 (30.3%) benign lesions. The average procedure time for MRI-guided needle localization was 32.9 minutes for a single site (range, 17–66 minutes) and 44.0 minutes for two sites (range, 28–66 minutes). In their study, pooled data from all reported MRI-guided localizations found 175/461 lesions to be malignant, with an overall PPV of 38% [68]. This is similar to MRI-guided biopsy. MRI-guided localization is therefore a procedure that should be used for lesions that are not amenable to MRI biopsy.

Challenges

The technical success rate of MRI breast biopsy is very high, reported between 95% and 100% [62]. Challenges to the MRI biopsy include the decreasing lesion conspicuity during the procedure (the so called "vanishing" target) and needle artifact obscuring the lesion site, with limitations in confirming lesion retrieval [8]. The "vanishing target" phenomenon was described for lesions that occurred when the lesion could no longer be well depicted during the procedure, due to the rapid washout of contrast in malignant lesions, accompanied by the progressive accumulation of contrast in the surrounding parenchyma (Fig. 5.10). The biopsy needle may often obscure lesions. Some centers solved this by additional injections of contrast material during the biopsy [32]. This is not a standard practice and generally is not required. Patient movement during the biopsy also results in misregistration and non-visualization of the lesion, if relying on subtraction of the contrast-enhanced from non-contrast sequences (Fig. 5.16). Some imaging protocols for MRI-guided interventional protocols may incorporate both fat suppression and subtraction and motion-correction software to reducing artifacts encountered with image subtraction [7].

Challenging Locations in MRI Biopsy

1. Lesions Close to the Nipple

(a) The retroareolar location is one of the most challenging locations for MRI breast biopsy. Changing the position of the tissue by rolling it may help, but this is challenging before injection of the contrast. Angling the needle and approaching the lesions from posterior to the lesions are generally most helpful to sample retroareolar lesions. Foam pads may be taped to the breast to support the retroareolar area within the compression plates [69]. Manual counter pressure may also be applied to the medial aspect of the breast by the radiologist while inserting the trocar and plastic introducer. This can avoid tenting of the skin or movement of the breast.

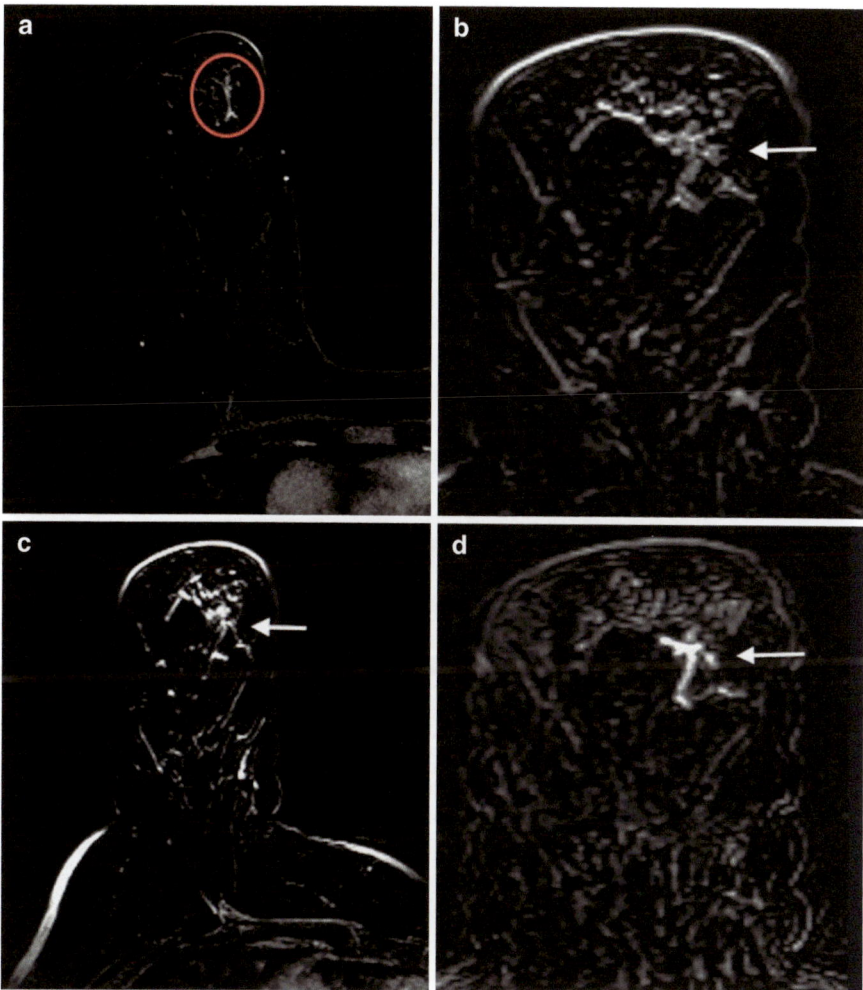

Fig. 5.16 (**a**) Enlarging linear branching non-mass enhancement in the retroareolar region of a 59-year-old woman being treated for locally advanced ipsilateral breast cancer. (**b**) MRI biopsy 2 weeks later 2 minutes and (**c**) 4 minutes post-contrast shows poor visualization of the NME. (**d**) A repeat subtracted contrast-enhanced image 6 minutes postinjection without motion better characterizes the best site to target for biopsy. Pathology results were invasive ductal carcinoma ER PR positive Her2 negative

2. **Lesions Close to the Chest Wall or Breast Implants**

For lesions that are very posterior in the breast, there are several possible solutions:

(a) One is the freehand technique first described by Daniel et al. where if the entrance point is located outside of the grid, the procedure can be performed unguided using an oblique path (Figs. 5.2 and 5.17). This can also

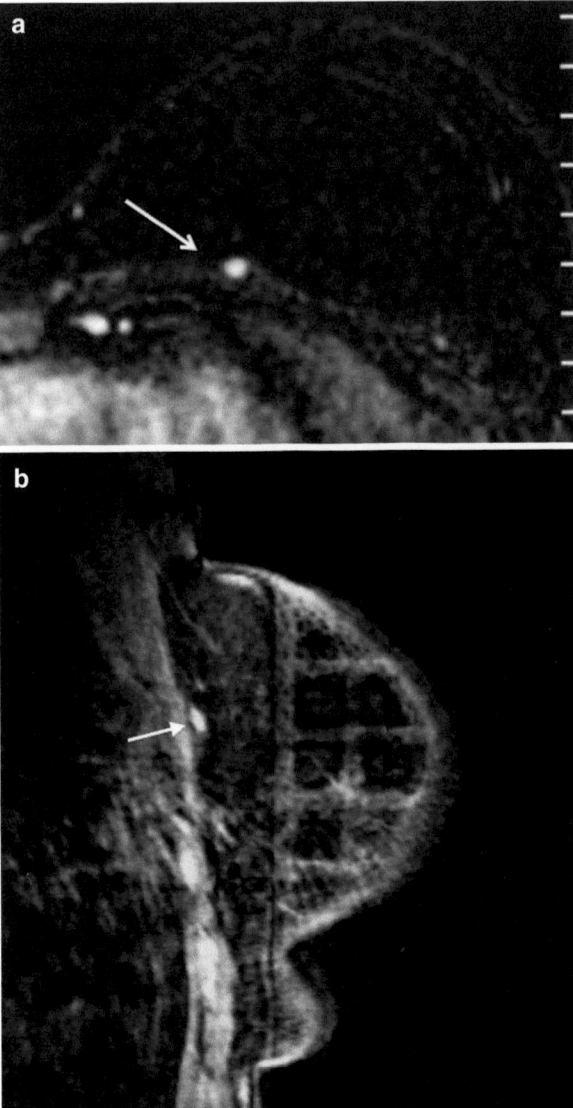

Fig. 5.17 A 58-year-old female with previous history of left lobular carcinoma treated by lumpec-tomy presented with chest pain, and (**a**) MRI showed a suspicious enhancing focus within the pectoralis muscle on axial subtracted T1 axial post-gad image. (**b**) Lesion is shown to be situated posterior to the compression plate and grid on sagittal T1 fat-suppressed sequence. (**c**) Needle was carefully angled posteriorly and confirmed to be in good position on axial T1 fat-suppressed image. (**d**) Post-biopsy sagittal sequence shows accurate sampling of the mass, and pathology confirmed a recurrent invasive lobular carcinoma. There were no complications of the biopsy due to careful technique used. This technique should only be used by experienced radiologists, and the patient could otherwise be managed with MRI-guided localization

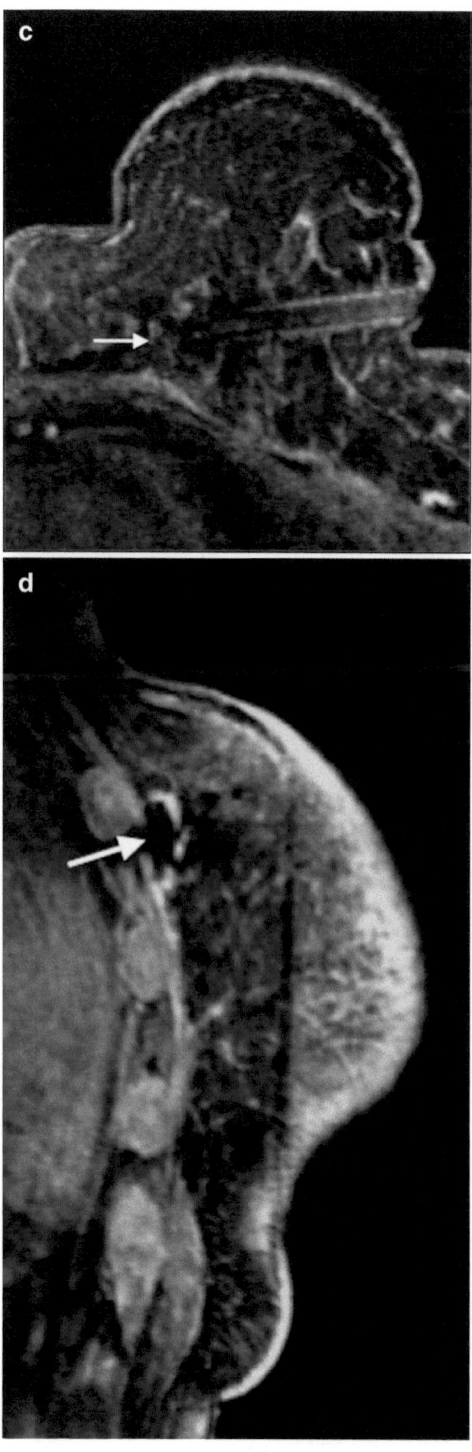

Fig. 5.17 (continued)

be used for lesions in the anterior part of the breast (Fig. 5.18) [56].
Although the cannula can be inserted at an angle, careful calculation of the
depth of the needle is required as this carries a risk of wall damage (pneumothorax, etc.)

(b) Some coils (Sentinelle) allow the grid to be shifted or moved (Fig. 5.13e).
    This technique may be used in cases where the lesion is posterior to the grid.
(c) For posterior medial lesions, the patient may be shifted to the contralateral
    breast coil opening and positioned in a semi-oblique position, permitting
    lateral access to the medial lesion [70].
(d) Removing the padding under the patient, bringing the patient's arm down by
    her side, and relaxing the pectoralis muscle as well as reducing the

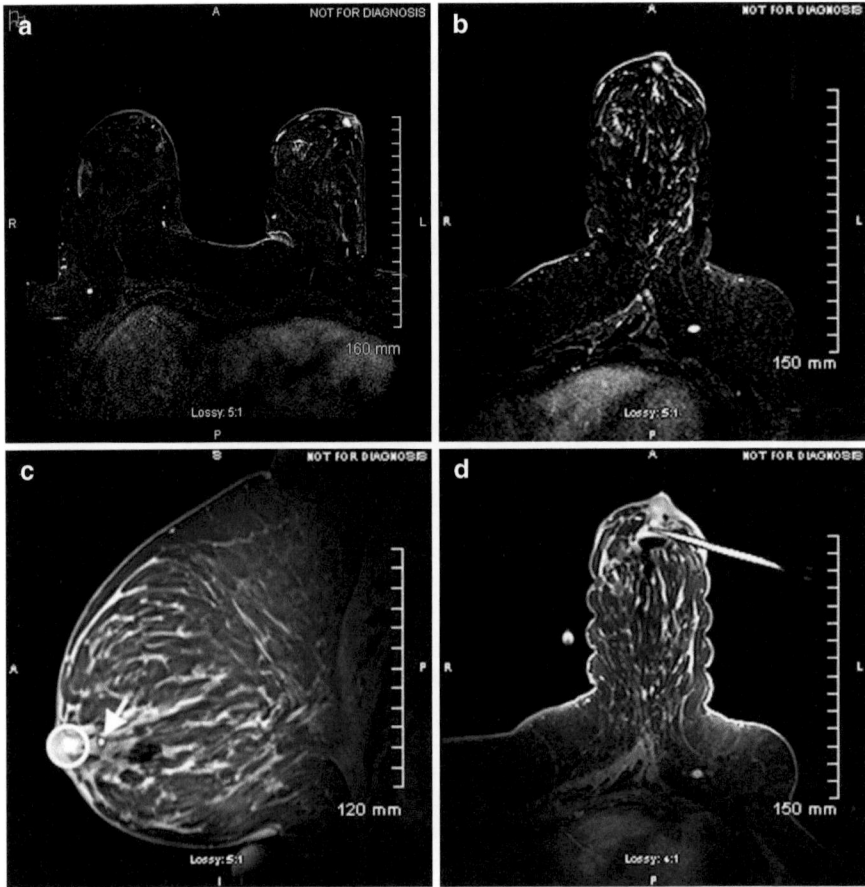

Fig. 5.18 Patient with nipple discharge and left retroareolar mass on (**a**) subtracted T1 axial post-
gad image. No US or MG correlate was found. (**b**) At MRI biopsy subtracted T1 axial post-gad
image shows persistent mass. (**c**) Sagittal T1 fat-suppressed image shows that mass (circle) is 1 cm
anterior to obturator (arrow). (**d**) Angled biopsy needle allows accurate sampling of the mass,
confirmed sclerosed papilloma with no atypia at pathology, and was almost completely removed
on 6-month follow-up MRI. (**e**) Axial T1 post-contrast subtracted image of retroareolar mass, with
signal void at clip indicating biopsy site (arrow)

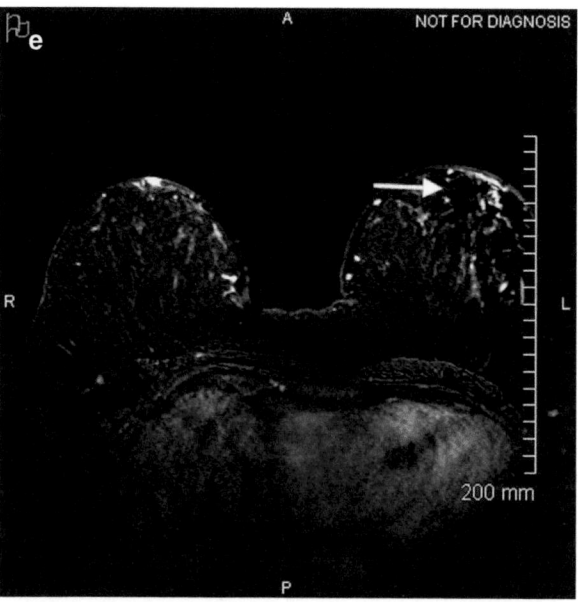

Fig. 5.18 (continued)

compression on the breast in the grid are techniques that may allow closer access to many posterior lesions.

(e) For medial posterior lesions, approaching the lesion from a lateral approach is generally required (Fig. 5.19).

(f) For lesions that are simply not safely accessible due to extremely posterior location, consideration should be made to deposition of a marker clip that can be localized for localization and surgical excision.

3. **Lesions Close to the Skin Surface**

(a) A minimum distance is required between the skin and lesion. If the lesion is too close to the skin surface, the skin may be damaged during sampling. To avoid this, a "half window" may be selected on the sampling device, which limits the sampling to the deeper part of the sampling trough and minimizes damage to the skin. This ensures that the sampling chamber is full in the breast and avoids the skin trauma of the cutting motion from sampling.

(b) For medial lesions close to the skin surface that are approached from the lateral side, a blunt tip needle may be selected to avoid damage to the skin (Fig. 5.19).

4. **Thin Breast**

(a) The minimum thickness is 30 mm for a standard needle and 18 mm with a shortened sampling chamber needle [71]. Local anesthetic may be injected into the breast parenchyma to increase the thickness of the breast by several mms [71]. The breast may be rolled to bolster the breast in thickness, and sponges may be used to support the breast.

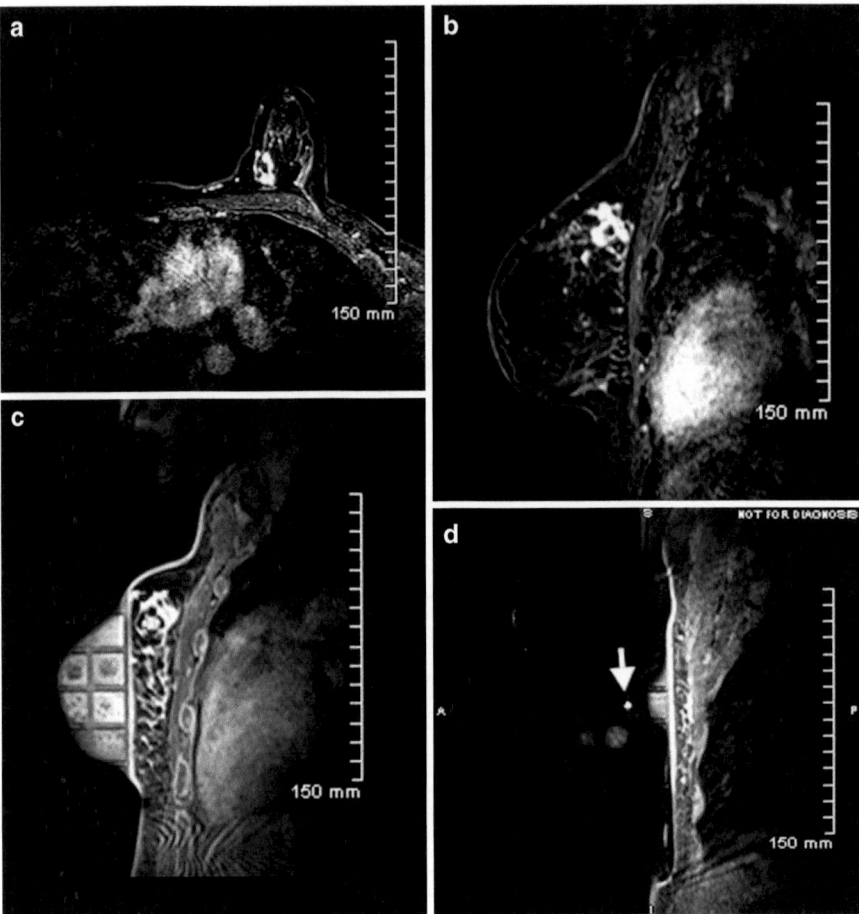

Fig. 5.19 A 38-year-old who underwent high-risk breast MRI screening showed a new 2.4 × 2.0 cm area of clumped heterogeneous NME. Second-look US and mammogram were negative, and MRI biopsy was recommended. (**a**) Axial T1 and (**b**) sagittal post-contrast subtracted images at time of MRI biopsy show the lesion to be posterior and medial in the left breast. (**c**) The lesion is posterior to the compression plate and grid in the medial breast. (**d**) The grid could only be used for needle placement (arrow) using a lateral approach. (**e**) The obturator is shown almost touching the skin medially and required a blunt tip needle for sampling. No complication of skin damage was found. The pathology results were sclerosing adenosis. This was considered discordant, and a repeat MRI biopsy was requested, but 6 weeks later (patient preference), (**f**) at repeat MRI biopsy, the lesion had resolved completely at the site of the signal void of the biopsy clip (arrow). Six-month follow-up MRI (not shown) confirmed the lesion had resolved

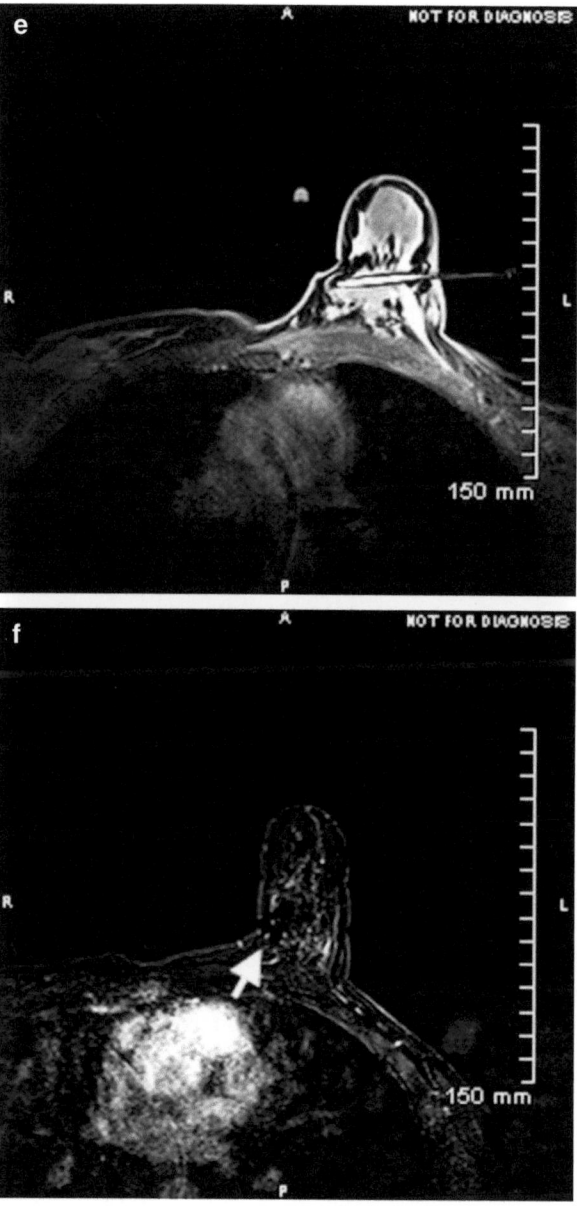

Fig. 5.19 (continued)

Needle Selection and Number of Samples

MRI biopsy should be performed with vacuum-assisted biopsy (VAB) instead of core needle biopsy (CNB) for several reasons, including lower upgrade rates, smaller lesions diagnosed at MRI, limitations of access and lack of continuous monitoring accurate targeting, shorter time and expense of MRI biopsy in repeat biopsies, and maximal diagnostic accuracy with VAB [6]. A minimum VAB needle size should be 11G.

Automated core biopsy requires that the needle must traverse a lesion to sample it. A vacuum-assisted biopsy needle may be placed *next* to the lesion and still acquire tissue from the lesion. This is the reason that vacuum-assisted biopsy is used over automated core biopsy [35]. Spick et al. reviewed the three different types of needle for VAB and found there was no significant difference between 8–10 VAB devices. Underestimation rates were similar between the three needles, and false negative rates were similar (1.1–5%) [72]. According to the European guideline, the minimum number of samples required with an 11G needle is 24 [73]. An equivalent volume may be taken with a larger gauge cannula, and the number of samples reported in the literature varies between 2 and 75 with a median of 12 [74].

Time to Perform the Biopsy and Number of Lesions

The first study by Lieberman on 20 women reported a mean of 35 minute (range 24–48 minute) for a single-lesion biopsy [35]. A subsequent study by Liberman et al. of 98 lesions biopsied found the median time to perform MRI-guided biopsy was 33 minute for one lesion and 56 minute for two lesions [75]. Lehman et al. reported that the average time to perform 19 single-site MRI-guided procedures was 38 minute (range, 23–57 minute) and biopsy of additional lesion(s) adds approximately 15–25 minute per patient [62]. No more than three lesions should be targeted, so as not to exceed the threshold for allowable local anesthetic. The average time in the MRI is approximately 1 hour, which increases by 30–50% when two or more sites are biopsied [74].

Sedation

Some centers may use sedation before the biopsy with benzodiazepines such as diazepam (Valium 1–2 mg oral doses, Roche Pharmaceuticals, Manatí, PR) or lorazepam (Ativan 1 or 2 0.5 mg oral dose or 5–10 mg intravenous dose, Wyeth-Ayerst Laboratories, Philadelphia, PA), on the morning of the procedure [35]. At our center, sedation is used with patients who are extremely anxious or claustrophobic. Patients must be gently sedated and awake for the procedure. However, the majority of patients do not require sedation and tolerate the procedure very well. It is essential that the radiologist communicate with the patient throughout the procedure, as this helps to reduce the patient's anxiety and encourages their cooperation during the biopsy.

Non-Visualization of Lesions at MRI Biopsy

In some circumstances, enhancing lesions will not be visualized on the day of the biopsy. This has been reported to range from 6.3% to 14.7% [33, 63, 75, 76]. First described by Kuhl et al. in 1997, it was identified that it was primarily due to excessive compression of the breast tissue [32]. To avoid non-enhancing targets, only gentle compression should be applied, enough to immobilize and stabilize the breast, not enough to prevent arterial blood flow. In most cases, it is due to resolved hormonally stimulated breast tissue (Fig. 5.9). A low rate of subsequent malignancy is reported to range from 0 to 10% [75, 76]. Therefore it is important to ensure a 6-month follow-up MRI for all non-visualized lesions to ensure that a malignancy is not missed.

Complications

MRI-guided VAB biopsy has very low rates of complications and morbidity, estimated between 0% and 6% similar to stereotactic breast biopsy. No complication is common [62]. Common complications include a small hematoma at the biopsy site, with infections rarely occurring. Patients should be warned of the possibility of a palpable lump at the biopsy site due to the hematoma, which may last several weeks. Other minor complications include malaise, pain, probe piercing the skin on the far side of the breast, and vasovagal reaction [60, 74, 75]. Careful biopsy planning and selection of the appropriate biopsy device should avoid skin damage. Good communication with the patient will usually ensure their collaboration to ensure an efficient and successful biopsy. Albeit very rare, it is conceivable that a pneumothorax could occur, and the radiologist should ensure that the freezing needle, trocar, and biopsy needle do not transgress the chest wall. Similarly, in the presence of breast implants, the possibility of implant rupture should be discussed with the patient before the biopsy. The possibilities of lesion non-visualization after contrast injection and undersampling of the lesion should be explained to the patient.

Clip Placement

Clips must be placed following MRI sampling and confirmed to be in the correct location post-biopsy. It is reported as correctly deployed in 93–100% of cases with failures due to bleeding or non-deployment in a superficial lesion, or a technical error [55, 75, 77].

Technical Issues

Radiologists must be particularly attuned to the ways in which the technical parameters of MRI biopsy affect evaluation of radiologic-pathologic correlation
(Fig. 5.20). The equipment used for an MRI biopsy uses field strengths of 1.5 or
3 T. Samples are taken outside the magnet to avoid image distortion and allow sufficient space. In general non-ferromagnetic tools are used, and careful attention is
paid to using any non-ferromagnetic equipment in the MRI suite to avoid accidents
(e.g., scalpels, needles, flashlights, etc.). Breast coils should allow external and
internal access to the breast. There are several different MRI vacuum-assisted
biopsy systems available, all of which use non-ferromagnetic material:

- Atec 9G (Hologic Inc., Bedford, MA).
- Vacora 10G (Bard Biopsy Systems, Tempe, AZ)

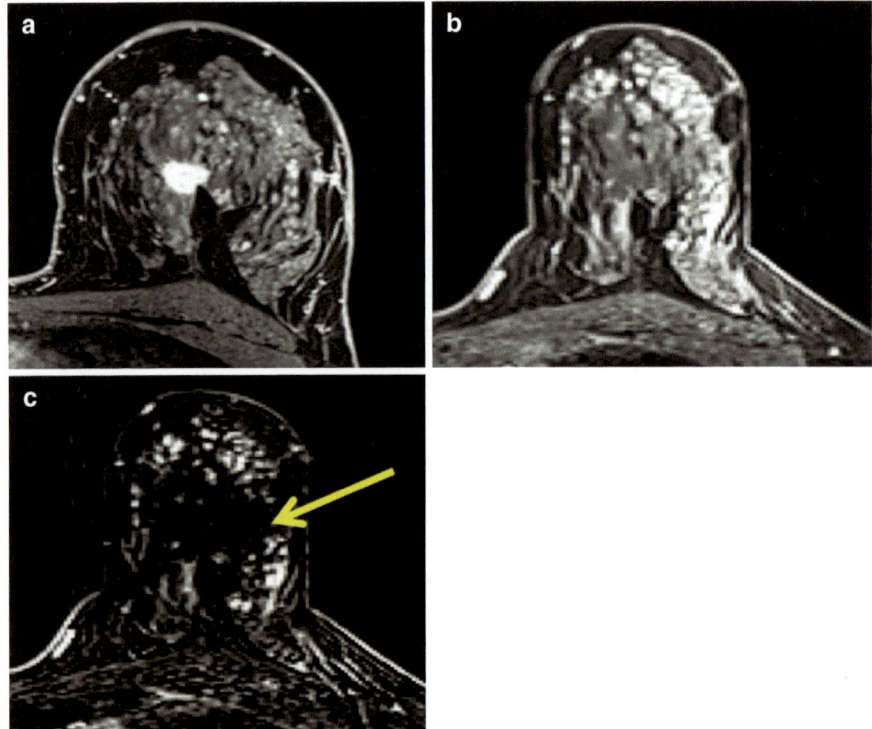

Fig. 5.20 (a) High-risk screening MRI identified a suspicious left enhancing mass on axial T1 contrast-enhanced fat-suppressed imaging for which no sonographic correlate was found. (b) The patient
returned 2 weeks later for MRI biopsy, but no enhancing mass was found on axial T1 post-contrast
images at the same location. (c) Subtracted T1 post-contrast imaging confirmed enhancement of the
remainder of the breast tissue. The signal void indicated a coil failure which was confirmed later due
to malfunctioning coil elements. The coil was replaced, and the patient returned 2 weeks later for
MRI biopsy (not shown) and was diagnosed with invasive ductal carcinoma at that site

- Senorx 10G (Bard Biopsy Systems, Tempe, AZ)
- Mammotome 11G (Devicor Medical Products, Cincinnati, OH)

Radiologic-Pathologic Concordance

As with any image-guided breast biopsy, but in particular with MRI biopsy, radiological-pathological concordance is of critical importance. The ACR Practice Parameter for MRI breast biopsies states that "the physician who performs the MRI-guided biopsy or presurgical needle localization procedure (or a qualified physician-designee) is responsible for obtaining results of the histopathologic sampling to determine if the lesion has been adequately biopsied and is concordant or discordant with the imaging findings" [7]. The results must be communicated to the referring physician and documented in the final report. Upgrade rates to malignancy and false negatives at biopsy are slightly higher for MRI-guided biopsy than for stereotactic-guided biopsy and US-guided biopsy, which makes radiologic-pathologic review essential [78].

Technical success rates are 96–100% with 95% clip deployment. Because it is not feasible to assess real-time sampling of MRI lesions and because specimen radiography cannot verify lesion sampling, determination of correct lesion sampling after an MRI biopsy is difficult. It is therefore essential to ensure good radiological-pathological correlation after an MRI biopsy.

Benign Concordant MRI Biopsies

Benign pathology is reported in 18–74% of lesions biopsied with MRI guidance, depending on the population of patients studied [35, 62, 75, 79–81]. The malignancy rates are typically always greater than 20%, therefore justifying the MRI biopsies.

MRI after benign concordant MRI-guided biopsy has shown that 8–12% of targeted lesions were inadequately sampled and, of those inadequately sampled, malignancy was ultimately diagnosed in 14–18% with a false negative rate of MRI-guided biopsy of 0.9–2.4% [77, 82, 83]. In their study of 177 lesions with benign concordant histology, Li et al. found that follow-up imaging before 6 months did not detect the missed cancers and 2 of the 4 missed cancers were stable [77]. Hauth et al. found that 14% of lesions may be missed entirely at MRI biopsy when performing a follow-up MRI 24 hours after biopsy while successful in 86% (25/29 lesions), partially removing the lesion in 69% (20/29 lesions), and completely removing it in 14% (4/29) [63]. If suspected to be unsuccessful, a repeat biopsy should be performed, and in the study by Hauth, this was done within 2–4 days. There is considerable overlap in the morphologic features of benign and malignant lesions such that reliance on the imaging features to determine concordance may be limited.

The significance of a lesion being stable on follow-up imaging at 6 months is questionable. Cancers, which were missed on MRI-guided biopsy, usually do not demonstrate an appreciable change in size sooner than 6 months [84]. Cancers may remain stable over 11–26 months (Fig. 5.20) [77, 82, 83]. Some authors have proposed a 12-month follow-up as a better alternative to benign concordant biopsy [83]. In the Hayward et al. study of 611 MRI breast biopsies, 68% of patients were excluded from the study cohort, because of lack of MRI follow-up [82]. Other studies show compliance rates of 57–70% [77, 83, 85]. With improved patient compliance and insurance reimbursement, this is a strong argument in favor of a 12-month follow-up.

Key Points
- It is challenging to determine a false negative MRI biopsy because real-time evaluation of sampling is not feasible.
- It is the lesions that prove stable at initial follow-up MRI after MRI-guided biopsy that should be regarded with caution. They may indicate a missed cancer.

Benign concordant pathology results may be categorized as specific or nonspecific [82]. Specific benign results include fibroadenoma, fat necrosis, pseudoangiomatous stromal hyperplasia (PASH), hemangioma, and lymph node. Nonspecific pathology results may include benign breast tissue, fibrocystic change, stromal fibrosis, fibrous tissue, usual ductal hyperplasia, apocrine metaplasia, and duct ectasia. In a study of 611 consecutive MRI biopsies by Hayward and colleagues, pathology of benign concordant biopsy was nonspecific in 70% (59/84) of cases, of which 41 were masses, 34 NME, and 9 foci [82]. At follow-up MRI obtained at an average of 10.5 month post-biopsy, the majority of lesions (75%) that underwent biopsy had resolved or decreased and supported a benign etiology [82]. *It is the lesions that prove stable at initial follow-up MRI that should be regarded with caution*; this may indicate that the lesions were not sampled at the time of biopsy and could represent a missed cancer (Figs. 5.21, 5.22 and 5.23). In the study by Li et al., 50% of the missed cancers were stable at initial MRI follow-up, and each of the missed cancers in the studies of Shaylor and Lee et al. was initially stable [77, 83, 86]. The initial follow-up MRI at 6 months may therefore help to recognize the need for rebiopsy and avoid delay in missed diagnosis of cancer. In a review of 85 benign concordant MRI lesions of patients who underwent follow-up MRI, a stable mass had a 25% probability of malignancy [85]. In this study, it was strongly recommended that a rebiopsy of a stable mass be considered, while NME could be followed with MRI without rebiopsy.

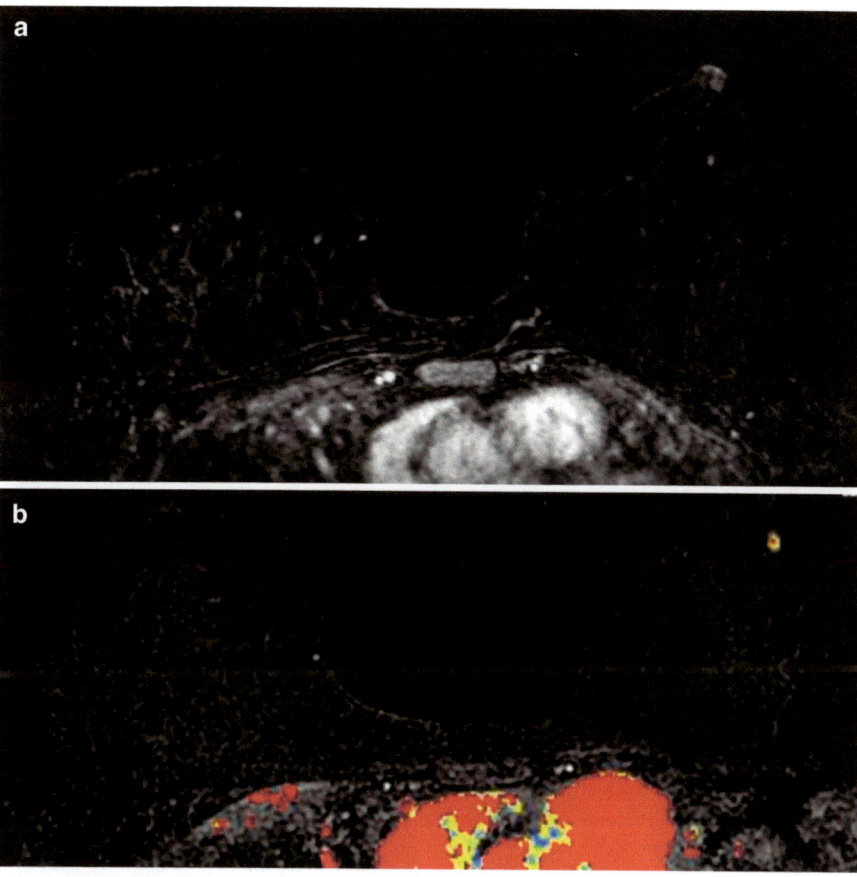

Fig. 5.21 Prior history of right breast cancer treated by lumpectomy for surveillance MRI. (**a**) Baseline MRI subtracted T1 axial 2 minutes post-contrast. A small focus in the retroareolar left breast is noted, called benign. (**b**) One year later, MRI shows interval increase in size of left retroareolar mass which demonstrates washout. An MRI biopsy was recommended. (**c**) Axial post-gad-enhanced subtracted images at day of MRI biopsy confirm presence of mass. (**d**) Sagittal T1 post-contrast image shows mass with suspicious features of rim enhancement. (**e**) Image of MRI biopsy done with angulation of the needle due to location of the lesion relative to the grid. (**f**) Sagittal image shows the obturator tip (short arrow) anterior to the enhancing lesion (long arrow). Eighteen cores of tissue were obtained with a 10 G VAB. Pathology results called benign mammary tissue with fibrocystic changes and columnar cell change, reported as concordant. (**g**) A 12-month follow-up MRI was done instead of recommended 6 months. No interval change was demonstrated, suggesting that the lesion had not been sampled. (**h**) A further 6-month follow-up MRI showed interval enlargement in the mass, prompting a repeat biopsy. Repeat biopsy axial (**i**) and (**j**) sagittal images post-sampling (36 cores) demonstrate no residual enhancing mass. Biopsy provided a diagnosis of periductal chronic inflammation and focal sclerosing adenosis. Surgical excision was recommended, which provided a diagnosis of intermediate nuclear grade DCIS. The mass had been relatively stable for 3 years, with two negative breast MRI biopsies

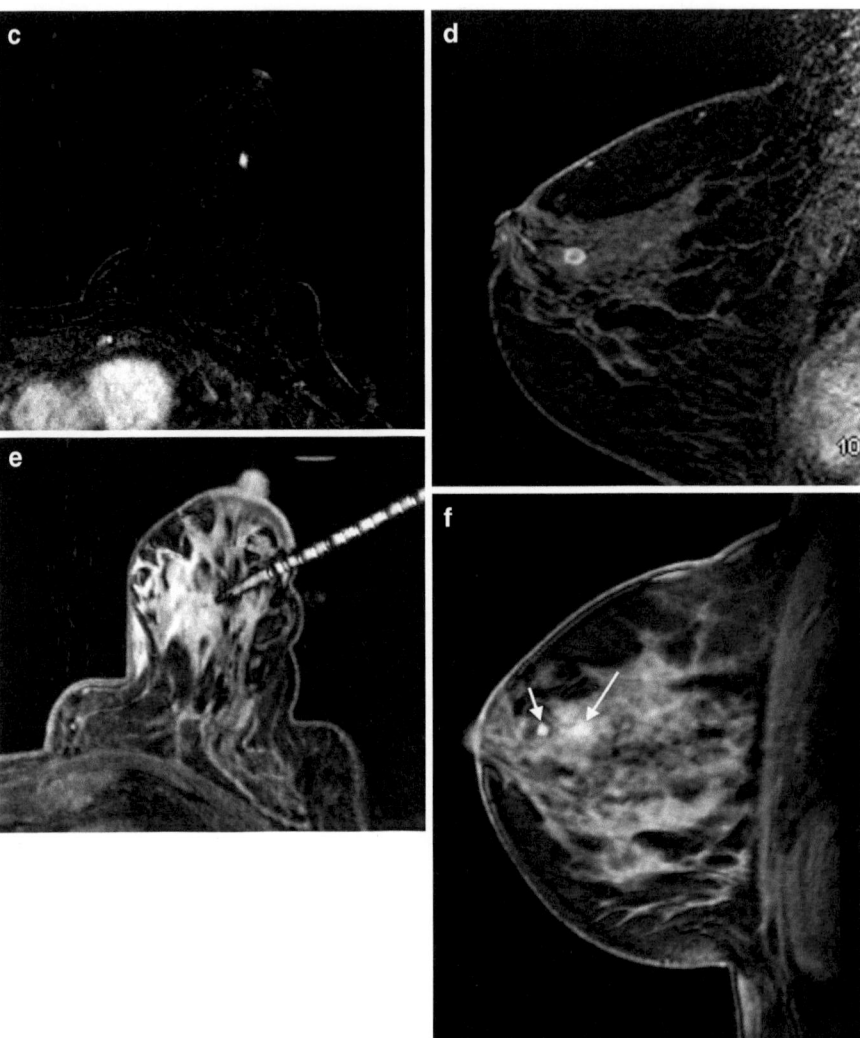

Fig. 5.21 (continued)

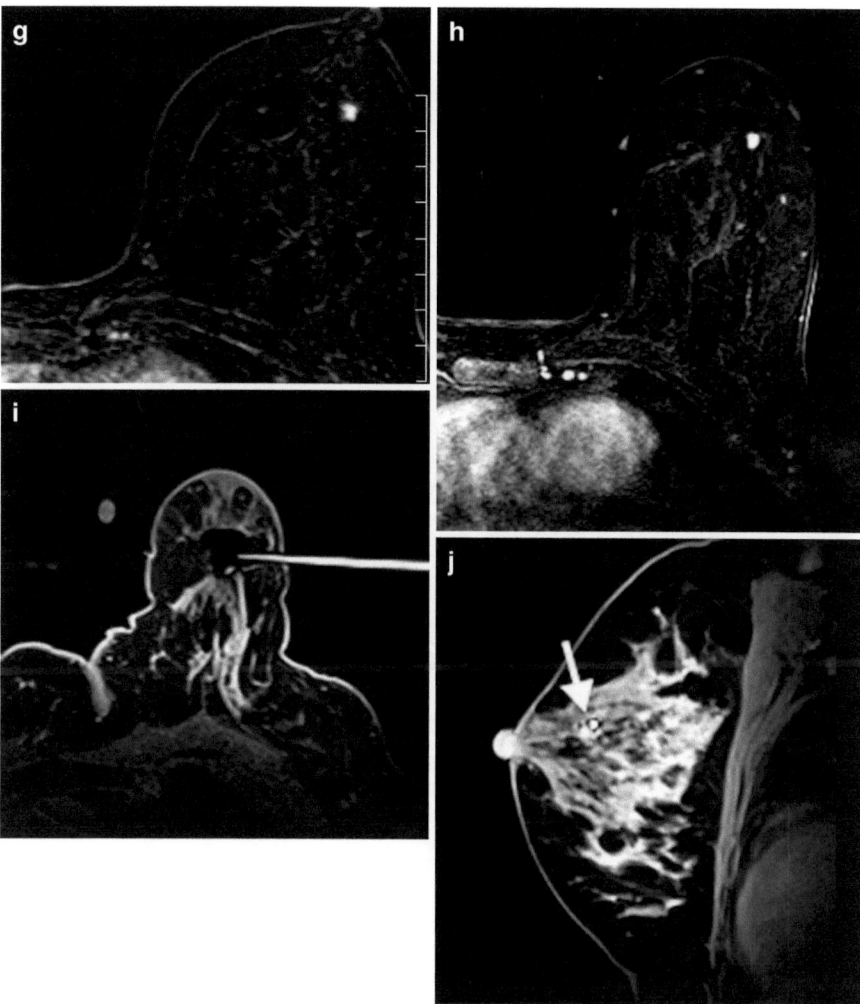

Fig. 5.21 (continued)

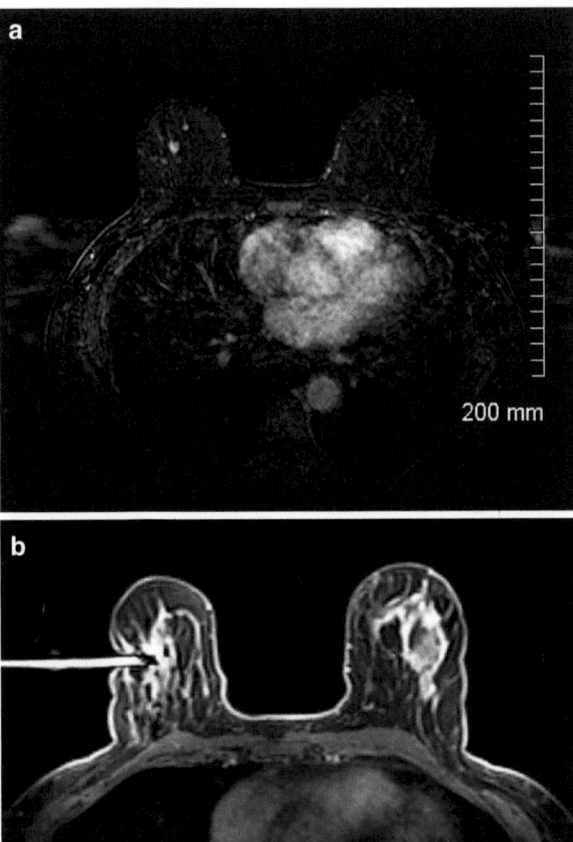

Fig. 5.22 A 66-year-old female with spontaneous clear left nipple discharge and normal mammograms and left breast ultrasound underwent problem-solving breast MRI. (**a**) Axial T1-weighted subtracted post-contrast image at 2 minutes shows a small 9 mm right enhancing mass with a possible non-enhancing septations and gradual (Type 1) kinetics. A second-look US was negative, and (**b**) MRI biopsy was performed, shown on axial and sagittal (**c**) images of the obturator in position posterior to the mass. A linear NME was also shown in the left breast (not shown), and MR biopsy for this lesion was also done. Pathology results were fibrocystic disease, proliferative with atypia and ductal ectasia, felt to be concordant with the findings. The left biopsy was consistent with a benign papilloma. (**d**) Follow-up breast MRI 6 months later showed the mass to be stable. The signal void (arrow) from the clip is posterior to the mass, suggesting in retrospect that the mass was not sampled. The patient was returned to routine screening mammography. (**e**) The patient presented 2 years later with metastatic lymphadenopathy to the neck and right axilla. Diagnostic CC (**f**) and MLO (**g**) right mammograms demonstrate a spiculated mass at the site of the previous right MRI biopsy (M clip). (**h**) Right breast ultrasound shows a poorly circumscribed mass at the location of the previous biopsy. Ultrasound-guided breast biopsy was consistent with invasive ductal and lobular carcinoma nuclear grade 2/3. Patient developed extensive bone metastases

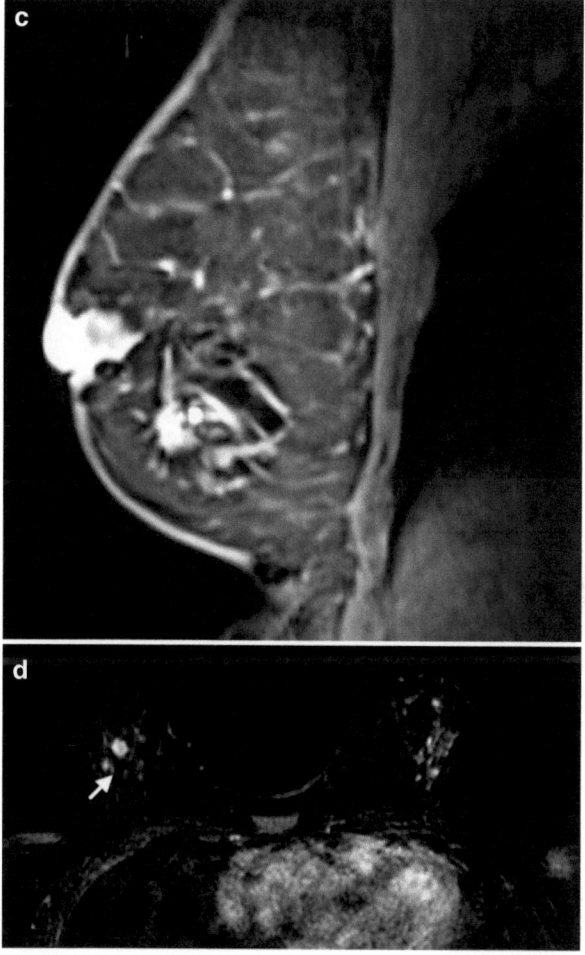

Fig. 5.22 (continued)

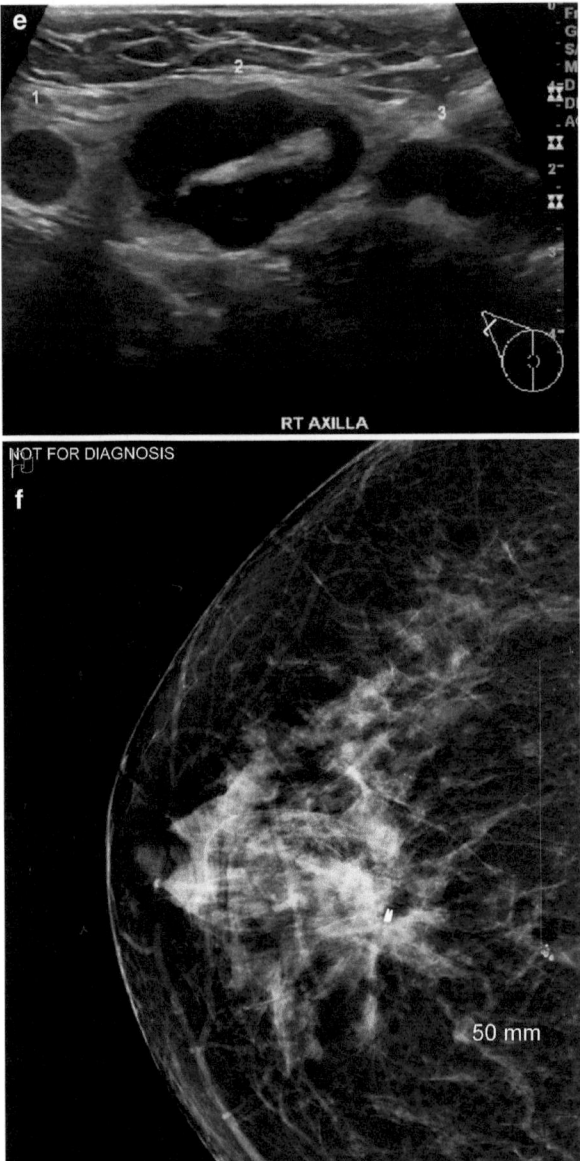

Fig. 5.22 (continued)

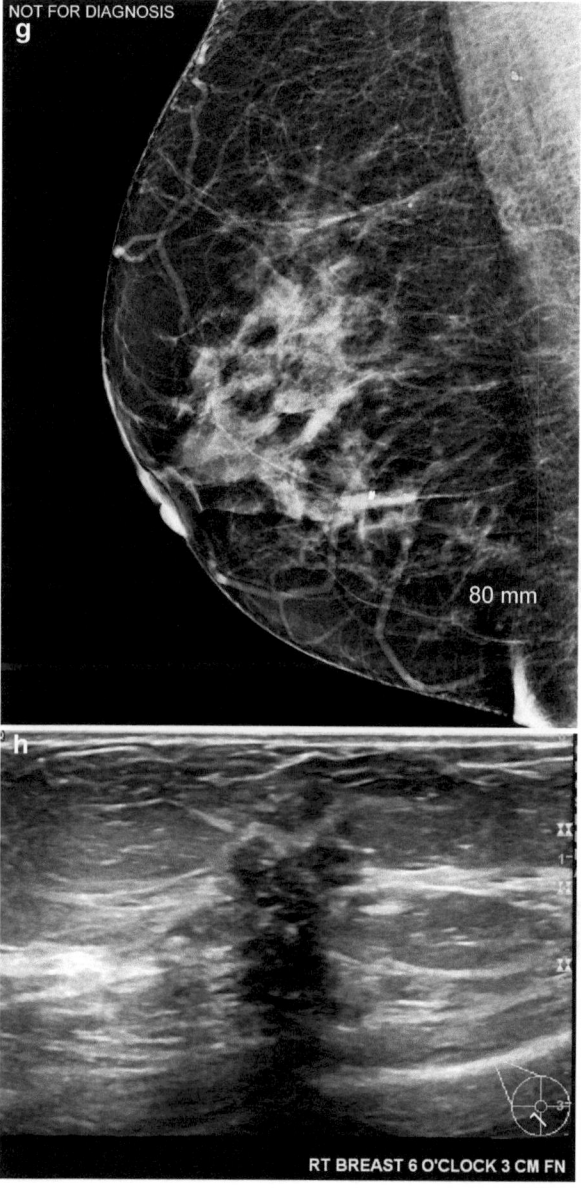

Fig. 5.22 (continued)

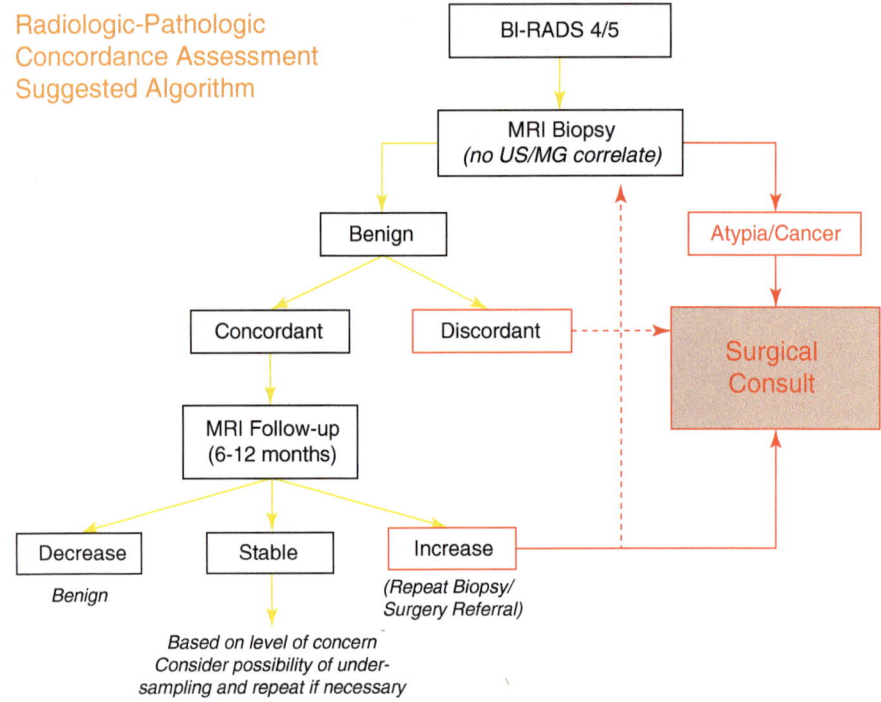

Radiologic-Pathologic
Concordance Assessment
Suggested Algorithm

Fig. 5.23 Suggested algorithm for radiologic-pathologic concordance of a BI-RADS 4 or 5 MRI-detected lesion

False Negative Rates

There are only a few small studies that report false negative rates, in the range of 0.9–2.3% [55, 77, 83]. In one of these studies, a single false negative biopsy was identified at 24 months following biopsy [83]. In the other study, 4 of 17 repeat biopsies of a total of 177 biopsied lesions were found to be malignant [77]. A recent larger study among 611 consecutive MR-guided breast biopsies at a single institution found a false negative rate of 2.4% [82]. In this study, two of the four carcinomas showed enlargement, one at 6 and the other at 12 months [77]. For this reason, authors suggest that MRI follow-up should be at 12 months instead of 6 months [83]. Regardless of whether the MRI follow-up is at 6 or 12 months, a follow-up MRI after a benign concordant MRI biopsy is essential to avoid a false negative MRI biopsy. In fact, continued MRI follow-up for at least 2 years is warranted in stable lesions given the small but definite risk of malignancy in long-term follow-up (see Fig. 5.21) [82].

Benign Discordant MRI Biopsies

Seven percent of all lesions are benign discordant pathology results at MRI biopsy, and 30% of benign discordant lesions undergoing surgical excision will prove to be malignant [86].

In one study of 342 MRI biopsied lesions, a significantly higher discordance rate was noted if the imaging target was missed rather than sampled, and a trend was noted toward a higher discordance rate in MRI lesions that were sampled rather than excised at MRI-guided vacuum-assisted biopsy [86]. They occurred more frequently in postmenopausal women and did not correlate with number of specimens obtained, indication for MRI, lesion type, or operator experience [86].

This compares with 3% (range 1–8%) of discordant rates at stereotactic and sonographic-guided biopsy with a frequency of cancer at rebiopsy of 14% (range 0–100%) [87–91]. This is likely related to the fact that MRI cannot confirm specimen sampling as well as the fact that MRI is performed in higher-risk women. Complete removal of the MRI target may reduce the likelihood of discordance and decrease the rebiopsy rate [86]. However, even with complete removal, surgery reveals residual cancer in 33–63% [75, 92].

High-Risk Lesions

High-risk lesions detected at MRI are seen with increasing frequency and range in incidence from 3% to 21% [55, 58, 60, 61, 93–95]. The most common high-risk lesion is atypical ductal hyperplasia, with other lesions including atypical lobular hyperplasia, lobular carcinoma in situ, radial scar, and papilloma. Atypical lesions or high-risk lesions may be upgraded to malignancy at surgery 13–57% and must be excised [72, 94–97]. This is higher than that reported for stereotactic breast biopsy. In one series, 41.7% (5/12) lesions were upgraded to invasive cancer and 58.3% (7/12) to DCIS [95]. Another series showed that all cases were upgraded to DCIS [94], while the largest series by Heller of 147 lesions had 63% (19/30) lesions upgraded to DCIS and 36.6% (11/30) to invasive carcinoma. The highest upgrade rate of all high-risk lesions is with ADH. Of 147 excised high-risk lesions diagnosed on MRI biopsy, the upgrade rate was highest for atypical ductal hyperplasia (34%), lobular carcinoma in situ (26.7%), and radial scar (24%) compared with papillary lesions (6.7%) and atypical lobular hyperplasia (13.3%) [96]. In this series, there was a significantly higher risk that a high-risk lesion would be upgraded to malignancy if the current MRI-detected high-risk lesion was in the same breast as a previously identified cancer, recently diagnosed cancer, or a remotely previously identified high-risk lesion [96]. There are no specific imaging features that predict upgrade for high-risk lesions when detected with MRI [95, 97].

Audits

Audits are strongly recommended [6, 7]. Performance benchmarks for breast MRI have been included in the BI-RADS lexicon, fifth edition [98]. These include CDR (20–30/1000), PPV3 (20–50%), sensitivity (>80%), and specificity (85–90%) percentage of minimal cancer (>50%) and node-negative invasive cancers (>80%). Rates for the performance for breast MRI screening in the community practice in the Breast Cancer Surveillance Consortium (BCSC) have also been published [99]. It is very useful for individual practices to audit their practices and to compare their performance with these benchmarks as a way of improving outcomes.

Acknowledgment *Acknowledgment for the help with figures is given to Dr. Raman Verma and Dr. Marina Mohallem-Fonseca of The Ottawa Hospital.*

References

1. Peters NH, Borel Rinkes IH, Zuithoff NP, Mali WP, Moons KG, Peeters PH. Meta-analysis of MR imaging in the diagnosis of breast lesions. Radiology. 2008;246(1):116–24.
2. Kuhl C, Weigel S, Schrading S, et al. Prospective multicenter cohort study to refine management recommendations for women at elevated familial risk of breast cancer: the EVA trial. J Clin Oncol. 2010;28(9):1450–7.
3. Sardanelli F, Podo F, Santoro F, et al. Multicenter surveillance of women at high genetic breast cancer risk using mammography, ultrasonography, and contrast-enhanced magnetic resonance imaging (the high breast cancer risk Italian 1 study): final results. Investig Radiol. 2011;46(2):94–105.
4. Mann RM, Kuhl CK, Kinkel K, Boetes C. Breast MRI: guidelines from the European Society of Breast Imaging. Eur Radiol. 2008;18(7):1307–18.
5. Kuhl CK, Strobel K, Bieling H, Leutner C, Schild HH, Schrading S. Supplemental Breast MR Imaging Screening of Women with Average Risk of Breast Cancer. Radiology. 2017;283(2):361–70.
6. Heywang-Kobrunner SH, Sinnatamby R, Lebeau A, Lebrecht A, Britton PD, Schreer I. Interdisciplinary consensus on the uses and technique of MR-guided vacuum-assisted breast biopsy (VAB): results of a European consensus meeting. Eur J Radiol. 2009;72(2):289–94.
7. American College of R. ACR practice parameter for the performance of magnetic resonance imaging -Guided breast interventional procedures; 2016.
8. American College of R. ACR practice parameter for the performance of contrast -Enhanced Magnetic Resonance Imaging (MRI) of the breast; 2018.
9. Berg WA, Zhang Z, Lehrer D, et al. Detection of breast cancer with addition of annual screening ultrasound or a single screening MRI to mammography in women with elevated breast cancer risk. JAMA. 2012;307(13):1394–404.
10. Kriege M, Brekelmans CT, Boetes C, et al. Efficacy of MRI and mammography for breast-cancer screening in women with a familial or genetic predisposition. N Engl J Med. 2004;351(5):427–37.
11. Leach MO, Boggis CR, Dixon AK, et al. Screening with magnetic resonance imaging and mammography of a UK population at high familial risk of breast cancer: a prospective multi-centre cohort study (MARIBS). Lancet. 2005;365(9473):1769–78.
12. Lehman CD, Blume JD, Weatherall P, et al. Screening women at high risk for breast cancer with mammography and magnetic resonance imaging. Cancer. 2005;103(9):1898–905.

13. Morris EA, Liberman L, Ballon DJ, et al. MRI of occult breast carcinoma in a high-risk population. AJR Am J Roentgenol. 2003;181(3):619–26.
14. Warner E, Plewes DB, Hill KA, et al. Surveillance of BRCA1 and BRCA2 mutation carriers with magnetic resonance imaging, ultrasound, mammography, and clinical breast examination. JAMA. 2004;292(11):1317–25.
15. Monticciolo DL, Newell MS, Moy L, Niell B, Monsees B, Sickles EA. Breast Cancer Screening in Women at Higher-Than-Average Risk: Recommendations From the ACR. J Am Coll Radiol. 2018;15(3. Pt A):408–14.
16. Fischer U, Kopka L, Grabbe E. Breast carcinoma: effect of preoperative contrast-enhanced MR imaging on the therapeutic approach. Radiology. 1999;213(3):881–8.
17. Hollingsworth AB, Stough RG, O'Dell CA, Brekke CE. Breast magnetic resonance imaging for preoperative locoregional staging. Am J Surg. 2008;196(3):389–97.
18. Lehman CD, Gatsonis C, Kuhl CK, et al. MRI evaluation of the contralateral breast in women with recently diagnosed breast cancer. N Engl J Med. 2007;356(13):1295–303.
19. Lee SG, Orel SG, Woo IJ, et al. MR imaging screening of the contralateral breast in patients with newly diagnosed breast cancer: preliminary results. Radiology. 2003;226(3):773–8.
20. Houssami N, Ciatto S, Macaskill P, et al. Accuracy and surgical impact of magnetic resonance imaging in breast cancer staging: systematic review and meta-analysis in detection of multifocal and multicentric cancer. J Clin Oncol. 2008;26(19):3248–58.
21. Lee CH, Smith RC, Levine JA, Troiano RN, Tocino I. Clinical usefulness of MR imaging of the breast in the evaluation of the problematic mammogram. AJR Am J Roentgenol. 1999;173(5):1323–9.
22. Moy L, Elias K, Patel V, et al. Is breast MRI helpful in the evaluation of inconclusive mammographic findings? AJR Am J Roentgenol. 2009;193(4):986–93.
23. Sardanelli F, Melani E, Ottonello C, et al. Magnetic resonance imaging of the breast in characterizing positive or uncertain mammographic findings. Cancer Detect Prev. 1998;22(1):39–42.
24. Bennani-Baiti B, Bennani-Baiti N, Baltzer PA. Diagnostic Performance of Breast Magnetic Resonance Imaging in Non-Calcified Equivocal Breast Findings: Results from a Systematic Review and Meta-Analysis. PLoS One. 2016;11(8):e0160346.
25. Sung JS, Lee CH, Morris EA, Comstock CE, Dershaw DD. Patient follow-up after concordant histologically benign imaging-guided biopsy of MRI-detected lesions. AJR Am J Roentgenol. 2012;198(6):1464–9.
26. Somerville P, Seifert PJ, Destounis SV, Murphy PF, Young W. Anticoagulation and bleeding risk after core needle biopsy. AJR Am J Roentgenol. 2008;191(4):1194–7.
27. Melotti MK, Berg WA. Core needle breast biopsy in patients undergoing anticoagulation therapy: preliminary results. AJR Am J Roentgenol. 2000;174(1):245–9.
28. Expert Panel on MRS, Kanal E, Barkovich AJ, et al. ACR guidance document on MR safe practices: 2013. J Magn Reson Imaging. 2013;37(3):501–30.
29. Heywang-Kobrunner SH, Huynh AT, Viehweg P, Hanke W, Requardt H, Paprosch I. Prototype breast coil for MR-guided needle localization. J Comput Assist Tomogr. 1994;18(6):876–81.
30. Coulthard A. Magnetic resonance imaging-guided pre-operative breast localization using a "freehand technique". Br J Radiol. 1996;69(821):482–3.
31. Orel SG, Schnall MD, Newman RW, Powell CM, Torosian MH, Rosato EF. MR imaging-guided localization and biopsy of breast lesions: initial experience. Radiology. 1994;193(1):97–102.
32. Kuhl CK, Elevelt A, Leutner CC, Gieseke J, Pakos E, Schild HH. Interventional breast MR imaging: clinical use of a stereotactic localization and biopsy device. Radiology. 1997;204(3):667–75.
33. Kuhl CK, Morakkabati N, Leutner CC, Schmiedel A, Wardelmann E, Schild HH. MR imaging--guided large-core (14-gauge) needle biopsy of small lesions visible at breast MR imaging alone. Radiology. 2001;220(1):31–9.
34. Heywang-Kobrunner SH, Heinig A, Schaumloffel U, et al. MR-guided percutaneous excisional and incisional biopsy of breast lesions. Eur Radiol. 1999;9(8):1656–65.

35. Liberman L, Morris EA, Dershaw DD, Thornton CM, Van Zee KJ, Tan LK. Fast MRI-guided vacuum-assisted breast biopsy: initial experience. AJR Am J Roentgenol. 2003;181(5):1283–93.
36. Kuhl C. The current status of breast MR imaging. Part I. Choice of technique, image interpretation, diagnostic accuracy, and transfer to clinical practice. Radiology. 2007;244(2):356–78.
37. Orel SG, Schnall MD. MR imaging of the breast for the detection, diagnosis, and staging of breast cancer. Radiology. 2001;220(1):13–30.
38. Radiology ACo. American College of Radiology Breast Imaging Reporting and Data System Atlas (BI-RADS Atlas). Reston: American College of Radiology; 2013.
39. LaTrenta LR, Menell JH, Morris EA, Abramson AF, Dershaw DD, Liberman L. Breast lesions detected with MR imaging: utility and histopathologic importance of identification with US. Radiology. 2003;227(3):856–61.
40. Abe H, Schmidt RA, Shah RN, et al. MR-directed ("Second-Look") ultrasound examination for breast lesions detected initially on MRI: MR and sonographic findings. AJR Am J Roentgenol. 2010;194(2):370–7.
41. Destounis S, Arieno A, Somerville PA, et al. Community-based practice experience of unsuspected breast magnetic resonance imaging abnormalities evaluated with second-look sonography. J Ultrasound Med. 2009;28(10):1337–46.
42. Shin JH, Han BK, Choe YH, Ko K, Choi N. Targeted ultrasound for MR-detected lesions in breast cancer patients. Korean J Radiol. 2007;8(6):475–83.
43. Wiratkapun C, Duke D, Nordmann AS, et al. Indeterminate or suspicious breast lesions detected initially with MR imaging: value of MRI-directed breast ultrasound. Acad Radiol. 2008;15(5):618–25.
44. Spick C, Baltzer PA. Diagnostic utility of second-look US for breast lesions identified at MR imaging: systematic review and meta-analysis. Radiology. 2014;273(2):401–9.
45. Meissnitzer M, Dershaw DD, Lee CH, Morris EA. Targeted ultrasound of the breast in women with abnormal MRI findings for whom biopsy has been recommended. AJR Am J Roentgenol. 2009;193(4):1025–9.
46. Liberman L, Mason G, Morris EA, Dershaw DD. Does size matter? Positive predictive value of MRI-detected breast lesions as a function of lesion size. AJR Am J Roentgenol. 2006;186(2):426–30.
47. Carbonaro LA, Tannaphai P, Trimboli RM, Verardi N, Fedeli MP, Sardanelli F. Contrast enhanced breast MRI: spatial displacement from prone to supine patient's position. Preliminary results. Eur J Radiol. 2012;81(6):e771–4.
48. Thomassin-Naggara I, Trop I, Chopier J, et al. Nonmasslike enhancement at breast MR imaging: the added value of mammography and US for lesion categorization. Radiology. 2011;261(1):69–79.
49. Clauser P, Carbonaro LA, Pancot M, et al. Additional findings at preoperative breast MRI: the value of second-look digital breast tomosynthesis. Eur Radiol. 2015;25(10):2830–9.
50. Mariscotti G, Houssami N, Durando M, et al. Digital Breast Tomosynthesis (DBT) to Characterize MRI-Detected Additional Lesions Unidentified at Targeted Ultrasound in Newly Diagnosed Breast Cancer Patients. Eur Radiol. 2015;25(9):2673–81.
51. Monticciolo DL. Postbiopsy confirmation of MR-detected lesions biopsied using ultrasound. AJR Am J Roentgenol. 2012;198(6):W618–20.
52. Trop I, Labelle M, David J, Mayrand MH, Lalonde L. Second-look targeted studies after breast magnetic resonance imaging: practical tips to improve lesion identification. Curr Probl Diagn Radiol. 2010;39(5):200–11.
53. Park VY, Kim MJ, Kim EK, Moon HJ. Second-look US: how to find breast lesions with a suspicious MR imaging appearance. Radiographics. 2013;33(5):1361–75.
54. Lee AY, Nguyen VT, Arasu VA, et al. Sonographic-MRI Correlation After Percutaneous Sampling of Targeted Breast Ultrasound Lesions: Initial Experiences With Limited-Sequence Unenhanced MRI for Postprocedural Clip Localization. AJR Am J Roentgenol. 2018;210(4):927–34.
55. Orel SG, Rosen M, Mies C, Schnall MD. MR imaging-guided 9-gauge vacuum-assisted core-needle breast biopsy: initial experience. Radiology. 2006;238(1):54–61.

56. Daniel BL, Birdwell RL, Ikeda DM, et al. Breast lesion localization: a freehand, interactive MR imaging-guided technique. Radiology. 1998;207(2):455–63.
57. Chen X, Lehman CD, Dee KE. MRI-guided breast biopsy: clinical experience with 14-gauge stainless steel core biopsy needle. AJR Am J Roentgenol. 2004;182(4):1075–80.
58. Perlet C, Heywang-Kobrunner SH, Heinig A, et al. Magnetic resonance-guided, vacuum-assisted breast biopsy: results from a European multicenter study of 538 lesions. Cancer. 2006;106(5):982–90.
59. Lampe D, Hefler L, Alberich T, et al. The clinical value of preoperative wire localization of breast lesions by magnetic resonance imaging--a multicenter study. Breast Cancer Res Treat. 2002;75(2):175–9.
60. Malhaire C, El Khoury C, Thibault F, et al. Vacuum-assisted biopsies under MR guidance: results of 72 procedures. Eur Radiol. 2010;20(7):1554–62.
61. Rauch GM, Dogan BE, Smith TB, Liu P, Yang WT. Outcome analysis of 9-gauge MRI-guided vacuum-assisted core needle breast biopsies. AJR Am J Roentgenol. 2012;198(2):292–9.
62. Lehman CD, Deperi ER, Peacock S, McDonough MD, Demartini WB, Shook J. Clinical experience with MRI-guided vacuum-assisted breast biopsy. AJR Am J Roentgenol. 2005;184(6):1782–7.
63. Hauth EA, Jaeger HJ, Lubnau J, et al. MR-guided vacuum-assisted breast biopsy with a hand-held biopsy system: clinical experience and results in postinterventional MR mammography after 24 h. Eur Radiol. 2008;18(1):168–76.
64. Program NHSBCS. Technical guidelines for magnetic resonance imaging (MRI) for the surveillance of women at higher risk of developing breast cancer 2012; NHSBSP Publication No. 68. Available at: https://assets.publishing.service.gov.uk/government/uploads/system/uploads/attachment_data/file/439601/nhsbsp68.pdf. Accessed 1 Dec 2018.
65. Soo AE, Shelby RA, Miller LS, et al. Predictors of pain experienced by women during percutaneous imaging-guided breast biopsies. J Am Coll Radiol. 2014;11(7):709–16.
66. American College of R. ACR practice parameter for performing and Interpreting Magnetic Resonance Imaging (MRI); 2017.
67. Causer PA, Piron CA, Jong RA, et al. MR imaging-guided breast localization system with medial or lateral access. Radiology. 2006;240(2):369–79.
68. Gao Y, Bagadiya NR, Jardon ML, et al. Outcomes of Preoperative MRI-Guided Needle Localization of Nonpalpable Mammographically Occult Breast Lesions. AJR Am J Roentgenol. 2016;207(3):676–84.
69. Chevrier MC, David J, Khoury ME, Lalonde L, Labelle M, Trop I. Breast Biopsies Under Magnetic Resonance Imaging Guidance: Challenges of an Essential but Imperfect Technique. Curr Probl Diagn Radiol. 2016;45(3):193–204.
70. Mahoney MC, Newell MS. Breast intervention: how I do it. Radiology. 2013;268(1):12–24.
71. Giess CS, Yeh ED, Raza S, Birdwell RL. Background parenchymal enhancement at breast MR imaging: normal patterns, diagnostic challenges, and potential for false-positive and false-negative interpretation. Radiographics. 2014;34(1):234–47.
72. Spick C, Schernthaner M, Pinker K, et al. MR-guided vacuum-assisted breast biopsy of MRI-only lesions: a single center experience. Eur Radiol. 2016;26(11):3908–16.
73. Heywang-Kobrunner SH, Sinnatamby R, Lebeau A, et al. Interdisciplinary consensus on the uses and technique of MR-guided vacuum-assisted breast biopsy (VAB): results of a European consensus meeting. Eur J Radiol. 2009;72(2):289–94.
74. Plantade R, Thomassin-Naggara I. MRI vacuum-assisted breast biopsies. Diagn Interv Imaging. 2014;95(9):779–801.
75. Liberman L, Bracero N, Morris E, Thornton C, Dershaw DD. MRI-guided 9-gauge vacuum-assisted breast biopsy: initial clinical experience. AJR Am J Roentgenol. 2005;185(1):183–93.
76. Pinnamaneni N, Moy L, Gao Y, et al. Canceled MRI-guided Breast Biopsies Due to Nonvisualization: Follow-up and Outcomes. Acad Radiol. 2018;25(9):1101–10.
77. Li J, Dershaw DD, Lee CH, Kaplan J, Morris EA. MRI follow-up after concordant, histologically benign diagnosis of breast lesions sampled by MRI-guided biopsy. AJR Am J Roentgenol. 2009;193(3):850–5.

78. Imschweiler T, Haueisen H, Kampmann G, et al. MRI-guided vacuum-assisted breast biopsy: comparison with stereotactically guided and ultrasound-guided techniques. Eur Radiol. 2014;24(1):128–35.
79. Ghate SV, Rosen EL, Soo MS, Baker JA. MRI-guided vacuum-assisted breast biopsy with a handheld portable biopsy system. AJR Am J Roentgenol. 2006;186(6):1733–6.
80. Perlet C, Heinig A, Prat X, et al. Multicenter study for the evaluation of a dedicated biopsy device for MR-guided vacuum biopsy of the breast. Eur Radiol. 2002;12(6):1463–70.
81. Tozaki M, Yamashiro N, Sakamoto M, Sakamoto N, Mizuuchi N, Fukuma E. Magnetic resonance-guided vacuum-assisted breast biopsy: results in 100 Japanese women. Jpn J Radiol. 2010;28(7):527–33.
82. Hayward JH, Ray KM, Wisner DJ, Joe BN. Follow-up outcomes after benign concordant MRI-guided breast biopsy. Clin Imaging. 2016;40(5):1034–9.
83. Shaylor SD, Heller SL, Melsaether AN, et al. Short interval follow-up after a benign concordant MR-guided vacuum assisted breast biopsy--is it worthwhile? Eur Radiol. 2014;24(6):1176–85.
84. Lee CH, Dershaw DD, Kopans D, et al. Breast cancer screening with imaging: recommendations from the Society of Breast Imaging and the ACR on the use of mammography, breast MRI, breast ultrasound, and other technologies for the detection of clinically occult breast cancer. J Am Coll Radiol. 2010;7(1):18–27.
85. Lee SJ, Mahoney MC, Redus Z. The Management of Benign Concordant MRI-guided Brest Biopsies: Lessons Learned. Breast J. 2015;21(6):665–8.
86. Lee JM, Kaplan JB, Murray MP, et al. Imaging histologic discordance at MRI-guided 9-gauge vacuum-assisted breast biopsy. AJR Am J Roentgenol. 2007;189(4):852–9.
87. Philpotts LE, Hooley RJ, Lee CH. Comparison of automated versus vacuum-assisted biopsy methods for sonographically guided core biopsy of the breast. AJR Am J Roentgenol. 2003;180(2):347–51.
88. Parker SH, Klaus AJ, McWey PJ, et al. Sonographically guided directional vacuum-assisted breast biopsy using a handheld device. AJR Am J Roentgenol. 2001;177(2):405–8.
89. Meyer JE, Smith DN, Lester SC, et al. Large-needle core biopsy: nonmalignant breast abnormalities evaluated with surgical excision or repeat core biopsy. Radiology. 1998;206(3):717–20.
90. Liberman L, Drotman M, Morris EA, et al. Imaging-histologic discordance at percutaneous breast biopsy. Cancer. 2000;89(12):2538–46.
91. Philpotts LE, Shaheen NA, Carter D, Lange RC, Lee CH. Comparison of rebiopsy rates after stereotactic core needle biopsy of the breast with 11-gauge vacuum suction probe versus 14-gauge needle and automatic gun. AJR Am J Roentgenol. 1999;172(3):683–7.
92. Liberman L, Morris EA, Lee MJ, et al. Breast lesions detected on MR imaging: features and positive predictive value. AJR Am J Roentgenol. 2002;179(1):171–8.
93. Viehweg P, Bernerth T, Kiechle M, et al. MR-guided intervention in women with a family history of breast cancer. Eur J Radiol. 2006;57(1):81–9.
94. Liberman L, Holland AE, Marjan D, et al. Underestimation of atypical ductal hyperplasia at MRI-guided 9-gauge vacuum-assisted breast biopsy. AJR Am J Roentgenol. 2007;188(3):684–90.
95. Strigel RM, Eby PR, Demartini WB, et al. Frequency, upgrade rates, and characteristics of high-risk lesions initially identified with breast MRI. AJR Am J Roentgenol. 2010;195(3):792–8.
96. Heller SL, Elias K, Gupta A, Greenwood HI, Mercado CL, Moy L. Outcome of high-risk lesions at MRI-guided 9-gauge vacuum- assisted breast biopsy. AJR Am J Roentgenol. 2014;202(1):237–45.
97. Heller SL, Moy L. Imaging features and management of high-risk lesions on contrast-enhanced dynamic breast MRI. AJR Am J Roentgenol. 2012;198(2):249–55.
98. Sickles EA DOC. ACR BI-RADS follow-up and outcomes monitoring. 5th ed. ed. ACR BI-RADS atlas, breast imaging reporting and data system: American College of Radiology, Reston; 2013.
99. Lee JM, Ichikawa L, Valencia E, et al. Performance Benchmarks for Screening Breast MR Imaging in Community Practice. Radiology. 2017;285(1):44–52.

Chapter 6
Radiology-Pathology Correlation

Dag Pavic

Radiology-pathology (Rad-Path) correlation can be viewed as a conclusion of the diagnostic process in breast imaging. Simply put, in Rad-Path correlation, we, radiologists, reconcile pathological diagnosis with imaging appearance and clinical picture. Based on the interaction of these three elements, we make recommendation for patient management [1, 2].

We will start this review of Rad-Path correlation with tissue samples obtained at imaging-guided biopsy. We will describe handling of the samples before they are sent to pathology. Elements of the Rad-Path conference will then be described, followed by the analysis of possible scenarios which might be encountered in daily work, with reference to Breast Imaging Reporting and Data System (BI-RADS) Atlas fifth edition [3]. Safe practice will be presented, based on my experience as a dedicated breast radiologist in different work settings, including academic and private practices.

Tissue Samples

Tissue sampling is performed after the results of noninvasive diagnostic modalities and clinical picture indicate that the lesion has a significant likelihood of being malignant, over 2%. We can perform needle biopsy, to obtain histological diagnosis, or fine needle aspiration for cytological diagnosis [4].

In most cases of ultrasound-guided biopsy, samples are placed in 10% formalin immediately after being harvested, directly from the biopsy needle sampling notch. We use a separate, saline-filled 10 ml syringe with 20G needle to gently push or scrape the sample out of the sampling notch. In some cases, when the sample sticks

D. Pavic (✉)
Medical University of South Carolina, Charleston, SC, USA
e-mail: pavic@musc.edu

© Springer Nature Switzerland AG 2019
C. M. Kuzmiak (ed.), *Interventional Breast Procedures*,
https://doi.org/10.1007/978-3-030-13402-0_6

to the biopsy needle, we use saline in the syringe to flush the sample directly into the formalin container. The amount of saline used for flushing, and in effect added to formalin jar, should be kept to minimum. We have not experienced any problems using this technique, over number of years, using the 120 ml clear plastic containers, prefilled with 80 ml of 10% formalin.

For stereotactic-guided biopsies, we use 60 ml clear plastic containers, containing 30 ml of 10% formalin. There should be enough formalin in the jar to completely embed the samples, at least ten times more than the total volume of samples, some authors say. Since we routinely obtain four to six samples, 30 ml of formalin is more than adequate.

Container is than sealed and clearly marked with a sticker carrying patient's identifiers. It's a good practice to write a succinct sample description on this sticker, for example:

• "R breast U/S Bx," standing for "Right breast ultrasound-guided biopsy."

In case there are more jars, with different sets of samples from other breast lesions in the same patient, we write "A," "B," etc. on the sticker, on the container lid, and in pathology requisition slip. While it might sound excessive, such practice can act as a safety net geared against specimen loss and can facilitate handling in pathology department. It also helps to avoid confusion when reviewing pathology results of multiple lesions in the same breast, sampled at the same time, since these letters used for labeling will be mentioned in pathology report.

There is one exemption regarding tissue procurement routine. When the lesion has a differential diagnosis which includes lymphoma, samples will be subjected to flow cytometry. Therefore, they should be placed in saline or in special media like RPMI, avoiding tissue fixation in formalin.

With calcifications as a target, regardless of imaging modality used for the guidance, we routinely perform X-ray of the samples before putting them in formalin. The goal is to confirm presence of calcifications in the samples: to ensure that the samples are of diagnostic value [5]. In an ideal world, samples without calcifications would not have been taken in the first place. Once we find the calcifications on image, we mark their position on the sample itself, as a sign for pathologist.

Calcifications are most often sampled with vacuum-assisted needle, 9-gauge(G) being rather common needle size. Interestingly, there seems to be no increase in diagnostic accuracy when 9-G or 8-G needle is used, when compared to a smaller diameter, 11-G needle [6–9]. When calcifications are visible on ultrasound, 14-G spring-loaded biopsy needle can be used, admittedly with mixed results. It is better to use vacuum-assisted needle of larger diameter, regardless of guidance modality. Samples obtained using these needles are larger and rather uniform in size and shape, depending on breast composition and consistency at the targeted area but also on the biopsy technique, as detailed below.

Vacuum-assisted needles have directional capability. Sampling notch opens on the side of the needle. Its orientation is controlled with a knob marked in hours, like a clockface. Modern tethered vacuum-assisted biopsy needle is automated, and it keeps performing the same biopsy cycle as long as it is turned on.

1. Inner needle cylinder retracts back, very quickly, and uncovers the sampling notch, a longitudinal aperture on the outer needle surface, close to the needle tip.

- In that moment, tissue adjacent to the opened sampling notch is pulled in by applied vacuum (suction, actually).

2. Inner needle cylinder then rotates and goes forward, thus cutting the tissue cylinder which lays inside the needle's sampling notch – this action is easily recognized by its distinctive sound.

- As the inner needle goes forward, it closes the sampling notch, and vacuum pulls the sample back, toward the needle's handle, where it is caught by the wire mash in sample container.

Cycle is then repeated, as long as the needle is on.

If we wanted to sample just an area located adjacent to needle's sampling notch, for example, at 12 o'clock, we would not need to rotate the needle. In practice, we sample at clockface numbers within a quarter or half a circle. Sample notch orientation as well as the number of samples will depend on the relative position of calcifications to needle and on the size of targeted calcification group. We reserve sampling through the full circle around the needle for architectural distortion.

In order to obtain good samples, one should turn the sampling direction knob fast and right after the noise of forward going rotating inner needle ceases. In this way, at the moment the sampling notch opens, the tissue will be settled and pulled straight in, without any twisting forces which can result in crush artifact seen under microscope, unnecessary tissue trauma, and bleeding. Alternatively, one can turn off the biopsy needle after each sample is taken, and rotate the needle at their leisure. This is slower and more cumbersome technique but can be justified when sampling calcifications in linear distribution. In such a case, mark the target somewhere in the middle of the group. If on target, there will be calcifications on the opposite sides of the needle, for example, at around 12 o'clock and around 6 o'clock. To minimize trauma and obtain optimal number of representative samples, we would take one or two samples around 12 0'clock; then stop the needle; rotate the sampling aperture toward opposite side of needle, around 6 o'clock; and then take one or two samples from that area. If fast enough, one can turn the needle for half a circle without breaking the biopsy needle cycle at all.

There are biopsy systems on the market, where needle rotation control can be preset and automated, thus decreasing the need for operator's involvement once the sampling starts.

Resulting sample is in fact a thin cylinder of tissue, its diameter defined by needle gauge, and its length by the longitudinal dimension of the sampling notch. Exact position of calcifications within the tissue sample should be marked on the sample itself.

Use sample radiograph as a guide. There are different ways one can obtain sample radiographs: using special containers, in one or two projections, etc. We use Petri dish, as the cheapest and most versatile option (Fig. 6.1).

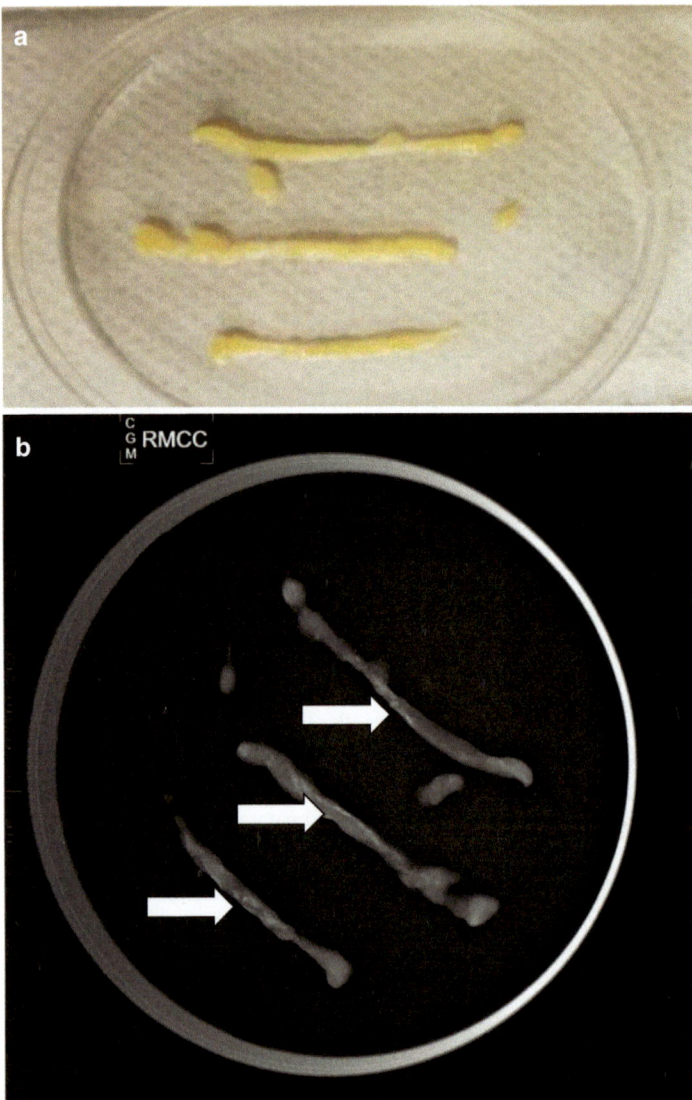

Fig. 6.1 Marking the location of targeted microcalcifications within stereotactic biopsy samples. Clinical: new, grouped amorphous microcalcifications. BI-RADS 4B. Tissue diagnosis: FCC with associated calcifications. Concordant. Recommended for 6-month follow-up unilateral diagnostic mammography. (**a**) Samples spread in Petri dish, extended to their full length and placed parallel to each other. Total of three samples were taken in this biopsy. (**b**) Sample radiograph, obtained using the magnification stand, confirms presence of microcalcifications, located centrally in each of three samples (white arrows). (**c**) We can manipulate sample radiograph on the workstation screen (rotate, flip vertically, flip horizontally, magnify, window/level) and/or rotate the Petri dish with actual samples, until they are matched, i.e., have the same left-to-right as well as top-to-bottom orientation. Then we look for calcification's position. In this case they are seen in the middle third of the sample (white arrow). We recognize their relation to the length, shape, and contours of the sample as seen on the radiograph and then find the same location on the real tissue. We mark it with tissue marking dye, using a swab. (**d**) Marked samples in Petri dish. Used swab is seen at the top. Samples will be placed in 10% formalin container and transferred to pathology

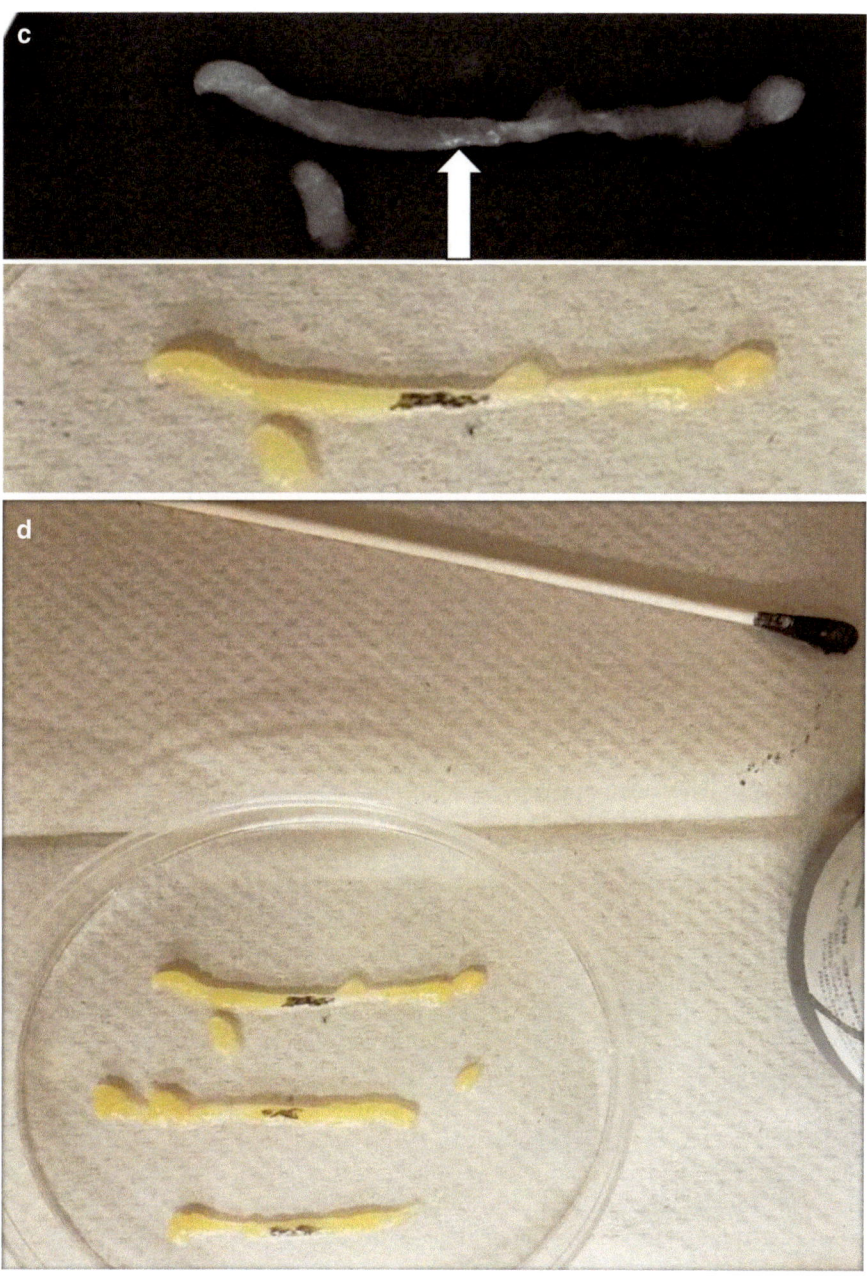

Fig. 6.1 (continued)

We transfer the samples from the container onto the Petri dish, trying to minimize the amount of fluid (saline, blood) in the dish. We might use the gauze pad to sop up the fluid from Petri dish, taking care not to touch the samples. Then we spread and separate samples in the dish, extend each one to its full length, and lay them more or less parallel to each other. Hence, we facilitate recognition of individual samples on the sample radiograph and make our job of marking the samples easier. We move samples around using the biopsy tools. They come handy, given that they were laid down on the biopsy tray after being used during the biopsy. Most often we use the lidocaine syringe with its needle, or a scalpel, or both. Given the sharpness of these tools, samples should be carefully manipulated to avoid crushing and slicing.

Sometimes samples are fragmented, and we are usually satisfied with just having them clearly separated, without trying to orient them in any special manner. We never leave the samples piled up onto each other before taking the sample radiograph.

Once the samples are conveniently spread on the Petri dish, we place it on magnification stand to achieve geometric magnification, thus improving depiction on resulting sample radiograph. In case calcifications are not clearly seen, change conditions (lower kV and increase mAs) and retake the image. In many cases calcifications can be seen better than on the prior diagnostic mammograms, when they were located within the breast. This is a chance to rethink our level of concern, i.e., designated BI-RADS assessment category.

When you look at samples, notice the position of calcifications relative to sample's length. When calcifications are in the middle of the tissue cylinder, that means the needle was at the optimal depth inside the breast, with the center of the sampling notch aligned with targeted calcifications. If calcifications are seen closer to the end of sample, we know that the Z coordinate, needle depth within the breast, was not optimal. This can be the end result of many factors: suboptimal targeting, too light compression, too much lidocaine injected into breast tissue between the skin entrance and target, plough effect of the needle, various mechanical factors (poor calibration, malfunction, etc.), and patient movement.

Of course, there are cases when calcifications are located close to the skin, and the only way to sample them is to modify Z coordinate intentionally, i.e., increase it for about 8 mm in typical case (1/3 of the needle's sampling notch length). In such a case, calcifications will be located close to the (proximal) end of the resulting sample.

We use tissue marking dye and long stem swabs to mark the samples. It is best not to use too much dye, as it can spread, stain the formalin in the jar, and can potentially adhere to sample in places we did not intend to mark. Once you dip the swab in the dye, remove the excess dye by swiping the swab tip against the inside walls of the dye bottle's neck.

We look at the samples using the radiograph as a guide: we want to match the real samples with the radiograph. We can flip the image horizontally or vertically on the workstation, and we can rotate Petri dish with samples, until they match each other. We look for the calcifications within the samples. When we locate some, we identify that individual sample in the Petri dish. Then we recognize local contours and shape of the sample, to find the exact spot on the real tissue. This point is lightly touched with the swab tip, to mark it for pathologist. When sample sticks to the swab tip, use a scalpel to gently separate them.

Once the calcifications are marked, samples can be transferred to formalin jar. They need to sit in formalin for 6–72 hours, in order to be fixed and ready for processing in pathology department.

There are newer, integrated biopsy solutions on the market today, where the samples are transported inside the biopsy needle from the sampling chamber into a special, compartmentalized sample container, being automatically separated from each other from the start. This container is then imaged, and compartments with samples containing calcifications are then marked (not samples themselves). The whole sample container is placed into provided formalin-filled jar, which is then sealed and is ready for transport to pathology. Such a system eliminates manual tissue handling in breast imaging department and protects the tissue from damage. Please note that in this case, the marked sample is not stained, and exact location of calcifications within the sample is not marked.

In any case, pathologist needs to know at least which was the sample, or samples, containing calcifications. In case we targeted calcifications, and they are not mentioned in pathology report, we will request to image the tissue blocks, to find calcifications (usually sparse) in the samples. The tissue block where calcifications are seen should be then imaged in orthogonal plane, to determine how deep within the tissue block they lay. Calcifications should be marked on the tissue block radiograph, to help pathologist. Additional deeper cuts of the tissue block, to the level where calcifications lay, will then be taken, processed, and examined in pathology again.

Samples are accompanied by a requisition slip. This is rare opportunity for a radiologist to take another role, to be an ordering physician. When we receive an order (e.g., for breast MRI), we appreciate every piece of information about the patient found in that order. Consequently, we will provide all the relevant information to pathologist in our requisition slip [1, 10].

First, we identify the source of samples by writing the lesion type and location, for example:

- "Calcifications. Right breast, 12 o'clock, middle depth."

Next, we list our differential diagnosis. For example, in case with grouped heterogeneous calcifications, it might look like:

- "FA, FCC, DCIS"

FA, fibroadenoma; FCC, fibrocystic changes; DCIS, ductal carcinoma in situ
Please note that the diagnoses are listed in their probability order, starting with the one which is most likely. In the above case, pathologist can clearly see what the radiologist expects the calcifications to be, most likely within FA, but they might also be within FCC or DCIS.

A succinct history can be of tremendous value to interpreting pathologist, sparing them the extra effort of looking for the patient's data in facility's health records. For example:

- "High-risk patient. Baseline mammography. R breast calcifications. BI-RADS 4B."

This is the perfect place and time to use proposed subdivision of BI-RADS 4 assessment category. Category 4 is very broad, covering more than 90% of all possible probability values, between 2% and 95%. By using a broad 4B category, radiologist misses the opportunity to effectively communicate with pathologist – he does not convey his level of suspicion based on imaging and clinical data. If he used subcategories, pathologist could easily recognize the assessed likelihood of malignancy:

4A   Low suspicion for malignancy (>2% to 10%)
4B   Intermediate suspicion (>10% to 50%)
4C   High suspicion for malignancy (>50% to <95%)

While the BI-RADS lexicon is clear, please note that Bi-RADS assessment category 5 (likelihood for malignancy 95% and more) reads "highly **suggestive** for malignancy," while 4C is "highly **suspicious**," to avoid possible confusion [3].

One should include a reasonable amount of pertinent data. Realistically, you are not going to write more than a dozen words or so. But bear in mind that pathologists are trained physicians who rely on clinical data, just as radiologists do.

Requisition slip is beginning of multidisciplinary interaction [11]. If our message to pathologist is clear, we can expect clear answer. One important detail: your writing should be legible.

Pathology requisition slip should include:

- *Lesion type*
- *Location*
- *Differential diagnosis*
- *BI-RADS category*
- *Brief history*

Reader might find interesting to go over an illustrated description of the sample's processing in pathology ward, from formalin jar to a finished slide (Fig. 6.2).

Pathology Report

Turnaround time for most of our biopsies is 1 or 2 business days, including Saturday. In some cases, more time is needed. When malignancy is encountered, in addition to microscopic histological examination, an immunohistochemical assessment is performed: typically, it includes estrogen and progesterone receptors and erythroblastic leukemia viral oncogene homolog 2 (ERBB2, formerly HER2/neu) protein expression [12].

Expression of Ki-67 protein, a cellular proliferation marker, is often routinely assessed immunohistochemically: it is used to distinguish luminal A and luminal B molecular subtypes of breast cancer and is positively associated with tumor grade.

Immunohistochemical profiling is clinically important as it represents the basis of molecular classification of breast tumors and has direct implications on breast

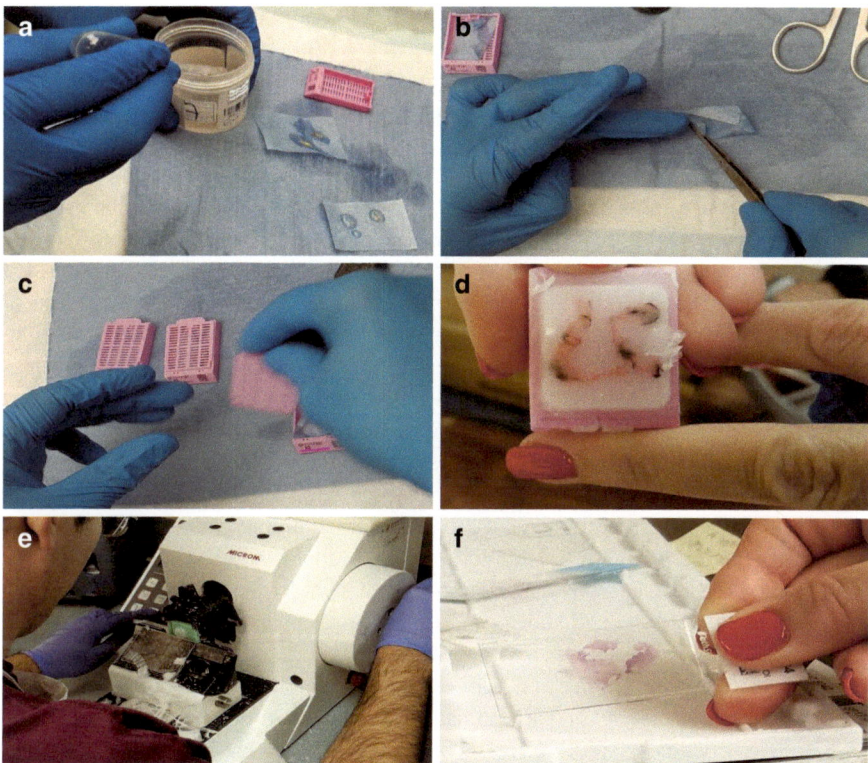

Fig. 6.2 Sample processing in pathology department. (**a**) Technologist uses pipette to transfer samples from container to filter paper. There is potential for losing some of the tissue at this step, especially with small, loose, mostly fatty tissue samples, which can stick to the sides of the jar. (**b**) Then he folds the paper and puts the enveloped sample into cassette, already engraved with patient's identifiers. (**c**) The cassette is then closed and is ready to be embedded in paraffin. (**d**) There is a resulting tissue block, with sample embedded in paraffin. Filter paper, used to wrap the sample, has been dissolved in the process (**e**) Tissue block is then cut on microtome, to the thickness of about 5 microns. Note that a number of slices from the very surface of the block are being discarded. Resulting thin slice is then taken with tweezers and placed on the glass to make a slide. (**f**) Slides are then stained and dried in semiautomated process and are ready for microscopic examination

cancer treatment choices in individual patient. However, for practical purposes, tumor markers do not play a significant role in Rad-Path correlation described here.

A typical pathology report consists of several components:

- Material received
- Findings

  - Most important finding or findings are listed first.
  - Other benign entities present in the samples, usually multiple.

- Summary and comment

In case there were multiple lesions biopsied in a single patient, it is of utmost importance to properly identify each lesion when learning about the pathology findings. That is the reason we labeled the samples from multiple lesions with "A," "B," and so on. When we include those labels in our requisition slip, they will be referenced in pathology report, making it easier to confidently identify each lesion.

Pathology report summary section might indicate diagnostic dilemmas, comment on the entity diagnosed, or even recommend complete excision of the sampled lesion, most often with incompletely sampled papillary lesions.

Please note that we tend to think of pathological diagnosis as of the final fact. While we must have a reference point, one should not forget that the pathological diagnosis is not unquestionable. Pathology, just like radiology, is based on observation. Observation boosted with counting and simple calculations, to be more precise. Any kind of observation, even one which includes quantification like counting the cell layers within a duct, is qualitative in nature and is more or less subjective. The results will depend on the observer's attention and experience, working environment, but also on the lesion's characteristics and the imaging modality used. This fact has long been recognized, both in radiology and in pathology.

Interobserver agreement in pathological evaluation of complicated cases can be significantly low, even among experienced breast pathologists. The same hematoxylin and eosin (H&E) stained slides can be diagnosed as usual ductal hyperplasia, a benign entity, atypical ductal hyperplasia (ADH), or even DCIS when read by different pathologists. Distinction between ADH and low-grade DCIS continues to be a diagnostic problem for pathologists, even with additional information from immunohistochemistry staining for surface antigens [13–15]. There are other significant entities which can present diagnostic problem for pathologists [16], including flat epithelial atypia (FEA) as well as cases of lobular neoplasia (LN): atypical lobular hyperplasia (ALH) and lobular carcinoma in situ (LCIS). Several of these entities can exist simultaneously and be present in tissue samples, complicating the situation even further.

Rad-Path Conference

In any case, with pathology report, it is time for Rad-Path conference. It can have different forms, from a single practitioner reviewing his biopsy results to a scheduled weekly conference with all breast radiologists and trainees present, such is the case in larger institutions.

Regardless of actual form, there is a shared essence: review the lesion's appearance, learn the pathological diagnosis, and recommend further management based on concordance between the two while considering lesion's likelihood of malignancy [1].

Rad-Path conference, being our last chance to catch cancer, is primarily geared toward improving patient care, but it should also be recognized as the prime educational opportunity. In short amount of time, a number of benign and malignant lesions are presented, described, categorized, and diagnosed, like in a case review exercise. If time and conditions permit, let the trainee review the images, describe the findings, and announce BI-RADS category prior to reading the pathology results, while the whole group reviews the images.

It is not too expensive to set a duplicate screen just for this purpose. We use a large diagonal flat screen television set which is connected to the workstation and set to clone display mode: it displays whatever is seen on diagnostic monitors. Image quality is non-diagnostic but is often sufficient, especially for ultrasound and MRI studies. Image quality can be improved by using preset, computer input picture mode on the television set and then by fine-tuning the image using brightness, contrast, hue, saturation, and other available controls, depending on television model. Having the ability to see the images, all participants in conference can test themselves on every case they were not involved with previously.

Each trainee should present several cases for the group. This exercise improves their ability to describe lesions using BI-RADS lexicon. While reviewing biopsy images, we use the opportunity to evaluate our biopsy technique and share individual experiences with different biopsy needles and other sampling tools.

We start with the prefilled list of patients who will be reviewed at conference. This list is prepared by trainees during the preceding week. We want to be time efficient, considering that the billable clinical work is at halt during conference. Having a list of patients instead of searching for individual patient in PACS during the conference saves precious minutes.

We review diagnostic images from the beginning of current encounter. In case of screening detected lesion, we start with screening mammogram and use prior exams for comparison. In cases which begun with clinical findings, like palpable mass, for example, brief pertinent history is presented.

We continue with review of diagnostic imaging: standard and additional mammography views and ultrasound in most cases. We describe the lesion or lesions, using BI-RADS lexicon. Our description leads to final BI-RADS assessment category. We already underlined usefulness of BI-RADS 4 subcategories.

Then we review biopsy images. We want to confirm that the lesion was properly sampled and that the samples were representative.

In ultrasound-guided biopsy, we first identify the targeted lesion and take two images in perpendicular planes, mimicking lesions appearance on diagnostic exam. We routinely record pre-fire image, depicting the targeted lesion and the biopsy needle with its tip positioned close to the lesion's margin. Next image is taken in post-fire needle position, showing the needle passing through the lesion. In some institutions short ultrasound video clips are taken and reviewed for this purpose.

The best way to confirm proper sampling with spring-loaded needle, in my opinion, is to use step-by-step biopsy technique and record three post-fire images (Fig. 6.3). In the first step, the inner stylet with a sampling notch is fired, and the sampling notch position is then adjusted, so it contains targeted lesion (or part of it). This relationship should be recorded on the first post-fire image. In the second step, outer needle is fired, and the second post-fire image is taken in the same plane, showing the biopsy needle and the targeted lesion. Ultrasound probe should then be

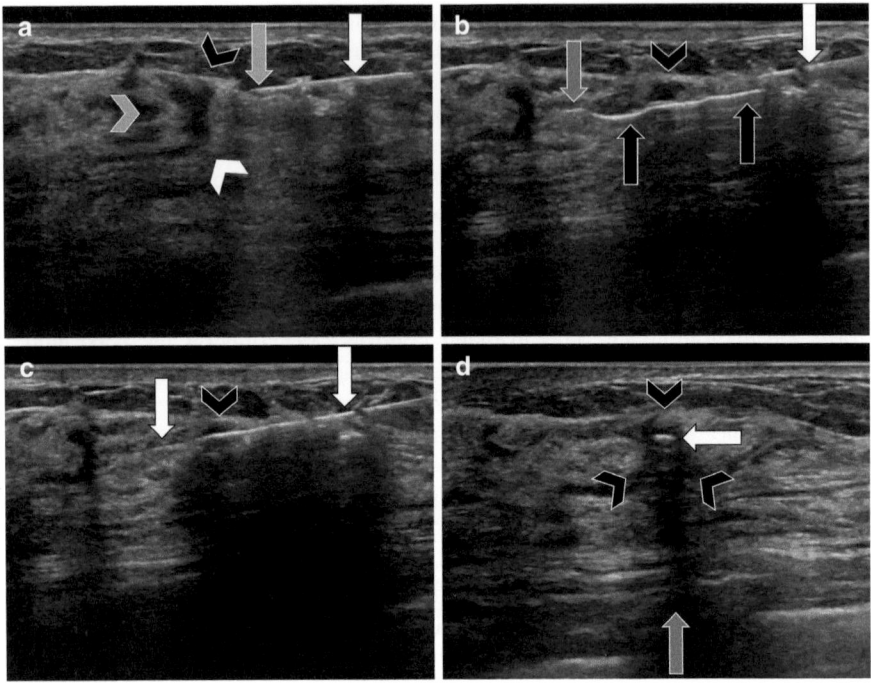

Fig. 6.3 Documentation of ultrasound-guided biopsy with a spring-loaded needle. Please note that resulting tissue sample has to fill at least two thirds of the sampling notch length, for these images unquestionably confirm proper sampling. Clinical: prior history of right breast LCIS, 6 years ago. Hypoechoic, irregular, nonparallel mass with spiculated border (gray arrowhead) with preserved ligament above it (black arrowhead), found on MRI directed ("second look") ultrasound of the left breast, not seen on breast tomography, BI-RADS 4B. Tissue diagnosis: stromal fibrosis, concordant. Follow-up ultrasound in 6 months. (**a**) Pre-fire image, showing the targeted hypoechoic mass in the image center (arrowheads), and the length of pre-cocked biopsy needle, seen as a straight reflector approaching from the right side toward image center (white arrow). The tip of the needle (gray arrow) is actually a part of the inner needle. It is seen in continuity with the outer needle (white arrow). To find the exact tip position, gently press the very end of the needle handle down: needle tip will point up. (**b**) First post-fire image, showing the fired stylet (inner part of the needle) position in relation to the targeted hypoechoic lesion, whose upper part is seen in the center of the image (black arrowhead). Outer part of the needle is still in original, cocked position, and is seen in the right side of the image as a straight reflector (white arrow). Where it stops, there starts another straight reflector, parallel to the first one but about 2 mm deeper (black arrows). This is the sampling notch of the inner needle. It traverses the targeted lesion and ends in a small hump, representing the needle tip (gray arrow). Note that this image was not taken immediately after the stylet was fired. Position of the sampling notch is adjusted, by moving the whole needle forward or backward, until the central part of the lesion can be seen around the sampling notch center. This relationship is then recorded, as seen on this image. (**c**) Second post-fire image, taken after the outer needle was fired, shows the outer needle (white arrows) traversing the lesion and covering the sampling notch. Only the topmost part of the targeted lesion (black arrowhead) remains visible above the needle. (**d**) Third post-fire image, taken in plane perpendicular to prior images, shows the needle in transverse section, seen as a 2–3 mm reflector (white arrow) with posterior shadowing (gray arrow), positioned within the bulk of the targeted lesion (black arrowheads)

twisted for 90 degrees, to take the final post-fire image in perpendicular plane, showing the needle in transverse section. Lesion-traversing needle would be seen as a shadowing, 2–3 mm hyperechoic reflector, located within the bulk of the lesion. Unfortunately, needle is sometimes seen off the target, adjacent to instead of within the lesion. Pathology results of such biopsy can be questioned, leading to the recommendation for repeat biopsy or surgical excision.

When biopsy targets suspicious calcifications, we look at sample radiograph to confirm the presence of targeted calcifications within samples.

At this point, pathology report is read. A verbatim read is the best approach, unless the one reading the report is experienced and can filter the report on fly, underlining important findings. Nowadays, pathology reports are increasingly structured, somewhat like ours. It becomes a matter of routine to quickly find information we are looking for, for example, was there a DCIS component in invasive carcinoma or whether calcifications were seen in samples.

This is the key moment in Rad-Path correlation. Pathology supplies the truth (within their limits) by listing the histologic entities diagnosed on tissue samples, and radiologists are matching that list with their own differential diagnosis which was based on imaging findings and clinical data. We will expand on this later in the text.

More often than not, results will be in concordance with our differential diagnosis and with the assigned BI-RADS assessment category, which we had duly entered in the requisition slip at the time of biopsy. We routinely accept such results without hesitation and recommend further management depending on underlying pathology and imaging findings. Often enough, though, pathological diagnosis can come as a surprise. Those cases will generally demand more time for evaluation.

It is possible to "cut corners" or, some may say, optimize the workflow in real-life settings. One may argue that those common benign cases with typical clinical presentation, like mobile, rubbery fibroadenomas in young patients, do not have to make it to weekly Rad-Path conference in busy practice. Such cases might be cleared by any breast radiologist in the group, without being reviewed by the whole group. We do not recommend such approach. In our practice, a single radiologist goes over all the biopsy results which were received during the day. He or she renders the results concordant or not and recommends management. This is a favored approach for many surgeons, because it helps to streamline their workflow and potentially speeds up the patient care. However, at our weekly Rad-Path conference, the group reviews all the cases from week before, for the final, group decision. In some cases, after thorough review and discussion, the group can make changes in management recommendation or even change the concordance designation rendered by a single radiologist. To avoid that scenario and potential confusion, in complicated cases or in cases with unexpected benign pathology results, no preliminary concordance is given before the group review. We always inform the surgeon of this situation as soon as it arises, so they do not expect our answer regarding concordance and management before Wednesday, when our weekly Rad-Path conference takes place.

When the group reaches consensus and makes recommendation for management, the diagnostic process is concluded, at least for the time being. Significant pathology results, concordance assessment, and group's recommendation are then recorded as an addendum to biopsy report. Final decision about patient management will be made at multidisciplinary conference, also known as breast tumor board, where all specialties involved in breast cancer patient care meet once a week and discuss each cancer case. Multidisciplinary interaction and exchange of information about the patient, integrating radiological, pathological, and clinical data, improves patient care [17–19]. In our practice, an attending breast radiologist and a breast imaging fellow participate in multidisciplinary breast conference which is held every week, day after our Rad-Path conference. Trainees are encouraged to attend this conference, as well. For some cases, usually those which are more complicated, radiologist would wait for multidisciplinary consensus before dictating addendum to biopsy report.

Breast radiologist participating at multidisciplinary conference should:

- Present images (including the staging studies) and describe imaging findings
- Announce discordant cases
- Recommend further imaging studies or procedures
- Answer imaging-related questions
- Actively participate in discussion

We must keep record of all the biopsies performed and their outcome, whether using a notebook or a computer program. This record is required in facility's audits mandated by Food and Drug Administration (FDA) and American College of Radiology (ACR) accreditation. On the side note, many breast imaging facilities utilize dedicated computer programs in daily work, from scheduling to reporting, in order to streamline their workflow but also to automatically collect data needed to satisfy audit requirements. Beside entering addendums to biopsy reports in patient's electronic health record, we keep a biopsy log in an old-fashioned, sturdy notebook. It helps trainees when presenting cases and can serve as a quick reference when clinician calls about random patient in the course of daily work, thus minimizing interruptions.

Our radiology nurse, more precisely breast imaging nurse, who brings us pathology reports on daily basis, participates in both Rad-Path and multidisciplinary conferences. She keeps her patient log and takes care of scheduling follow-up imaging and other recommended radiology procedures. She also tracks the patient at later time and ensures that they comply with recommended follow-up imaging.

Rad-Path Correlation

- Brief pertinent history.
- Review pre-biopsy imaging studies.
- Describe the lesion, develop differential diagnosis, and assign BI-RADS category.

- Confirm proper sampling.
- Learn the pathological diagnosis.
- Assess for concordance.
- Reconcile with clinical data.
- Recommend management.
- Dictate addendum to biopsy report.

Addendum to biopsy report

- Main pathological diagnosis
- Concordant or not
- Management recommendation

This concludes the description of Rad-Path conference. We will now expand on radiology-pathology concordance per se.

Rad-Path Correlation

Rad-Path concordance is defined in BI-RADS Atlas: "A tissue diagnosis is considered to be concordant if cytological or histological diagnosis rendered by the pathologist is consistent with the imaging findings of the biopsied lesion" [3].

Non-critical implementation of this rule in clinical practice would not result in optimal patient care. There is significant overlap in imaging appearance of benign and malignant entities across imaging modalities, and these entities can be present in the breast side by side, to complicate the matter. Supposedly pathognomonic appearance can be misleading: post-lumpectomy scar can look like cancer. Tissue diagnosis – biopsy – is a sampling procedure: we take only small amount of tissue, and even smaller amount of tissue is actually examined under the microscope. Every biopsy carries a risk of sampling error. The lesion itself can be heterogeneous, composed of varying components, which can be misleading for pathologist. Even with good, representative samples, accurate diagnosis is not certain. There are borderline lesions, those which present a diagnostic problem for pathologists. Therefore, accepting every concordant result as a sufficient premise for management recommendation is not the best option. Our judgment cannot rely only on imaging and pathology. We should, and we do include all available clinical data in the decision-making process.

There is multitude of possible scenarios which can be encountered in Rad-Path correlation. We already touched on some of them. In the Table 6.1 below, we present a simplified frame of reference using BI-RADS assessment category as the basis for Rad-Path correlation.

Table 6.1 Simplified Rad-Path correlation scenarios

Pathology	Radiology	Concordance	Management recommendation
Non-confirmatory	Any BI-RADS	Discordant	Repeat biopsy, surgical excision
Malignant	Any BI-RADS	Variable	Surgical excision
			Additional imaging, additional biopsy
Benign	BI-RADS 5	Discordant	Surgical excision
	BI-RADS 4C	Discordant[a]	Surgical excision, repeat biopsy
	BI-RADS 4B	Variable	To be discussed
	BI-RADS 4A	Concordant[b]	Imaging follow-up (routine or short term)
	BI-RADS 3	Concordant	Routine imaging follow-up
	BI-RADS 2	Concordant	Routine imaging follow-up

[a]In majority of cases
[b]In most cases

As it was stated previously, in Rad-Path correlation, we first want to confirm that the lesion recommended for biopsy was actually sampled (Fig. 6.4). For ultrasound-guided biopsy, we compare its sonographic appearance, size, and location with diagnostic ultrasound exam. Biopsy marker clip position on post-biopsy mammogram is also reviewed and compared to prior diagnostic imaging studies.

In cases with multiple biopsy clips in the same breast, their proper identification can be a daunting task. We use different clips in various shapes, to avoid confusion (Fig. 6.5). It is a good practice to label clips on images in PACS, using simple descriptors, like "old" (lesion) and (lesion) "A," "B," "FA," "FCC," "DCIS," and so on, as appropriate in particular case. It speeds up imaging review and makes it easier. For stereotactic-guided biopsy targeting calcifications, we look for the calcifications on sample radiograph first. Then we try to identify those same calcifications on prior diagnostic mammograms and correlate their location with the biopsy clip location on post-biopsy mammograms. In practice the biopsy clip can end up at distance from the biopsy area, as evident on post-biopsy mammograms [20]. Clip migration should be documented in the biopsy report, stating the distance and direction from the targeted lesion. When reviewing these images prior to preoperative needle localization, described clip migration must be considered.

Biopsy can be non-confirmatory: pathological diagnosis does not explain lesion's imaging appearance (Fig. 6.6). For example, pathological diagnosis of FA cannot explain palpable, spiculated mass with architectural distortion, highly suggestive for malignancy. In some cases, pathology will offer non-specific results, described as benign breast tissue, or there will be no breast tissue present in samples, at all. In both scenarios, such histology cannot explain lesion's imaging appearance, and it represents discordant result.

In these cases, we still want to obtain tissue diagnosis. We will recommend surgical excision when the lesion was properly sampled. In cases with questionable biopsy technique and when suspicious lesion was actually missed at biopsy, we might recommend repeat biopsy, instead [21].

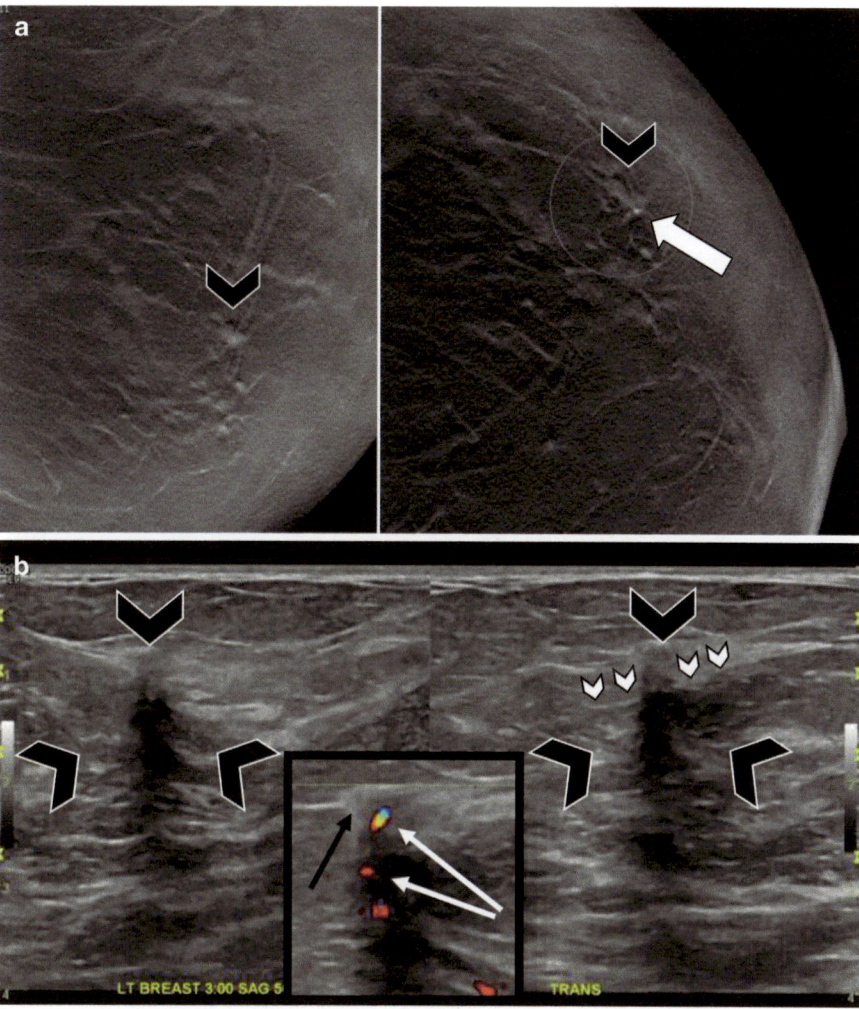

Fig. 6.4 Review of diagnostic and biopsy images. Clinical: postmenopausal female, status post right mastectomy for IDC. New mass with architectural distortion seen on annual tomography and confirmed on targeted US. BI-RADS 4C. (**a**) Breast tomography. Enlarged, 1 mm thick reconstructed slices in MLO and CC projection. Subcentimeter irregular isodense mass (black arrowhead) with associated single coarse microcalcification (white arrow) and architectural distortion in the central lateral breast, middle depth, at about 3 o'clock. (**b**) Targeted breast US. Hypoechoic, irregular, nonparallel, shadowing mass (black arrowheads), with non-circumscribed, angular margins and internal vascularity (white arrows, inset), breaking through the ligamental plane (white arrowheads). Note a thick hyperechoic border (not a BI-RADS descriptor), sign of infiltration (black arrow, inset). It is not possible to completely delineate the lesion: its deep border is not discernible due to shadowing. (**c**) Post-fire US image at US-guided biopsy. Needle (white arrows) is seen traversing the lesion (black arrowhead). Please note that the needle's echogenicity diminishes from right to left, toward the needle tip. The needle is positioned slightly off the image plane, and its tip position is not ascertained. (**d**) Post-biopsy mammograms in CC and ML projection, showing the clip position at the biopsy site (white arrows), in the same area where the lesion was seen on diagnostic tomography, confirming that the correct target was sampled

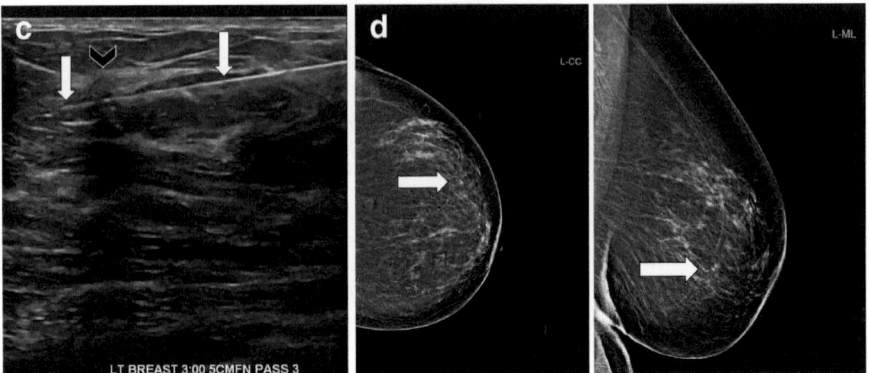

Fig. 6.4 (continued)

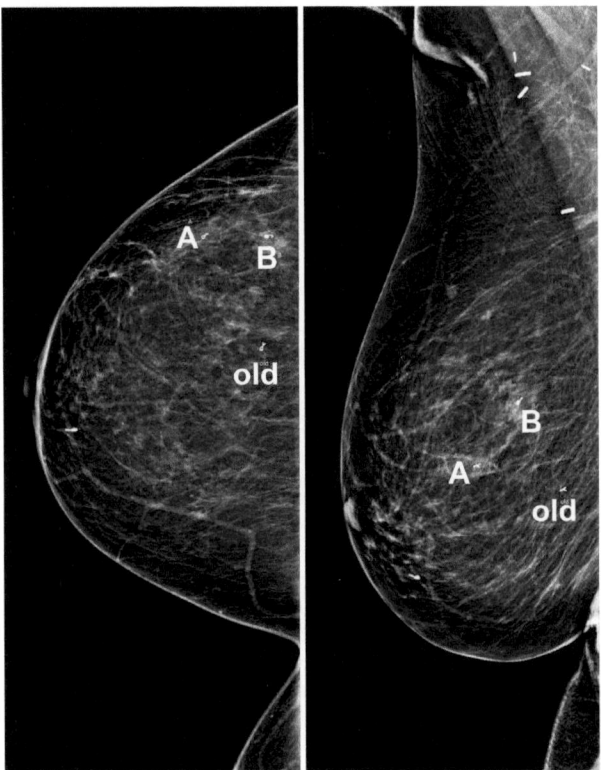

Fig. 6.5 Multiple clips labeled on radiographs for easier identification. Clinical: status post right lumpectomy and sentinel node excision, 3 years ago. Two new non-palpable masses in the upper outer quadrant found at annual breast tomography and confirmed on targeted US. BI-RADS 4C. Tissue diagnosis: IDC and IDC, both concordant. Recommended for surgical consult and excision. There are three biopsy marker clips in the right breast, seen on CC and ML post-biopsy mammograms. Two clips are similar looking, ribbon-shaped. The one located in central posterior breast is labeled "old," indicating that it is not a part of current patient encounter. Two clips located in central lateral breast, middle and posterior depth, were placed at the same time, serving as markers for targeted lesions labeled "A" and "B." Note: original labels are small, so they were enhanced for illustration purposes

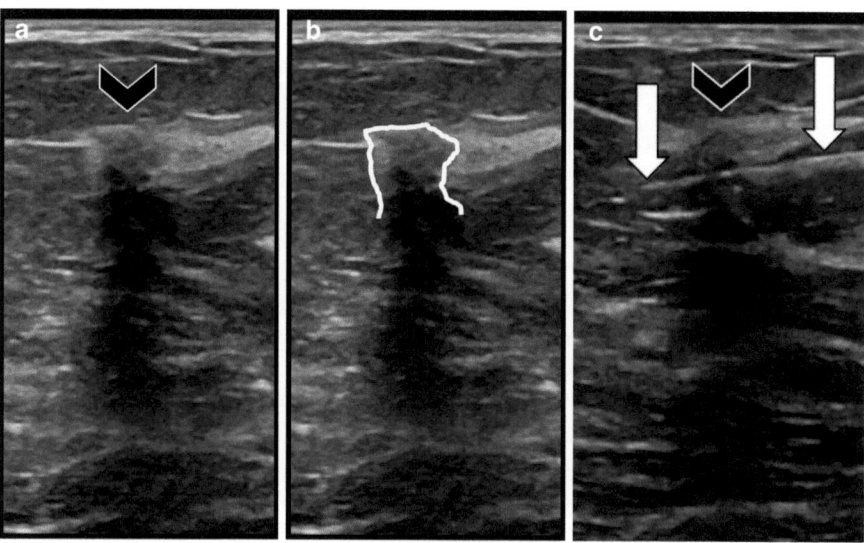

Fig. 6.6 Review of biopsy images after discordant pathology result. Clinical: same case as in Fig. 6.4. Postmenopausal female, status post right mastectomy for IDC. New mass with architectural distortion seen on annual tomography and confirmed on targeted US. BI-RADS 4C. Tissue diagnosis: fat necrosis and adipose tissue. Discordant. (**a**) US image of the same lesion as in Fig. 6.5 (black arrowhead). (**b**) The same US image with white contour line superimposed on the lesion. Note that the lesion's deep border cannot be delineated, as it is undistinguishable from posterior shadowing. (**c**) Needle (white arrows) is seen traversing the lesion (black arrowhead) on the post-biopsy image (on the right). However, it passes through the hypoechoic area, where lesion's deep border cannot be separated from shadowing. After learning about benign pathology result of fat necrosis and benign breast tissue, we considered the real possibility that the lesion, or at least its representative portion, was missed. Recommended for surgical excision. Final pathology: ILC, gr. 1

In our practice these scenarios occasionally happen, but we rarely recommend repeat biopsy of the same lesion. If lesion's location renders the biopsy technically difficult, it will be the same on repeated attempt, unless patient's positioning could have been remedied by some maneuver which was not exploited at the first biopsy. For example, in ultrasound-guided biopsy of lesion located in the lateral aspect of the breast, patient was not placed in the full lateral recumbent position to reduce lesion's apparent depth, resulting in more difficult biopsy.

Patient's preference should be taken into account at this point: Is she willing to go through another biopsy, which likely was not the most pleasant experience in the first place, or would she rather have surgical excision, possibly even in general anesthesia? A clinician, usually a surgeon, should be the one who can find answers to these questions and make the final decision.

Malignant pathological diagnosis at biopsy will invariably result in recommendation for surgical excision, whether we expected malignancy or not. Whenever we receive malignant pathology, we want to act fast, so we immediately notify breast surgeon about the results, even before the Rad-Path correlation takes place.

When malignancy was expected, we want to confirm that the lesion's size and location were correctly reported in prior diagnostic report, to ensure proper staging.

Also, we want to review diagnostic images, to search for additional significant lesions and/or exclude benign ones. Contralateral breast and ipsilateral axillary status are of particular importance for staging and management; therefore our recommendation might include additional imaging and even additional biopsy to exclude other possibly suspicious lesions prior to final treatment planning. For example, when DCIS is found on biopsy of suspicious calcifications, we might want to sample additional, similar looking group of calcifications at distance from the one sampled. The other possible strategy in such case might be to perform breast magnetic resonance imaging (MRI), which has high sensitivity for DCIS (depending on reader's experience and the amount of background parenchymal enhancement). MRI exam might be the preferred way to establish extent of disease since it will also detect potential lesions in the opposite breast. Decision between these two strategies will depend on multitude of factors but mainly on patient's and surgeon's preference. We communicate our recommendations at multidisciplinary breast conference. During multidisciplinary interaction, it can turn out that our management recommendation is not feasible. Surgeon might be aware that the patient had already decided to have mastectomy done, for example, and does not want to go along with our recommendation for additional biopsy to exclude multicentric disease.

In unexpected malignancies – lesions with low likelihood for malignancy on imaging but with positive biopsy results – the first thing we want to exclude is any error in sample identification, labeling, and transfer to pathology. These would be extremely rare but should be excluded, especially when dealing with multiple lesions in the same breast. Then, all available imaging studies should be meticulously reviewed in search for subtle findings which might have been overlooked initially but can be seen in malignancies, like the small segment of irregular margin of an otherwise circumscribed hypoechoic mass, for example. This is valuable opportunity for the whole group, especially for trainees, to sharpen their diagnostic skills. In these cases, additional imaging will often be recommended, MRI in particular, due to its high sensitivity.

Malignancy is sometimes an incidental finding, with no signs on imaging studies (Fig. 6.7). With category BI-RADS 4B microcalcifications as target, for example, pathology results might include FCC with associated calcifications, what is concordant with the imaging appearance, but listed in report as one of the benign entities after the primary diagnosis of intermediate-grade DCIS without associated microcalcifications, which is mammographically occult disease.

When we accept the fact that virtually all lesions with malignant results on biopsy will be recommended for surgical excision, Rad-Path correlation can be reduced to a single question: Can we accept benign results?

Given that the lesion is properly identified, benign pathology result is acceptable when it satisfies two conditions:

1. Lesion's imaging characteristics match the known imaging appearance of one or more benign entities in pathology report – pathology is concordant according to BI-RADS Atlas.
2. Lesion's assessed likelihood of malignancy, expressed through the BI-RADS assessment category, is low enough in our judgment.

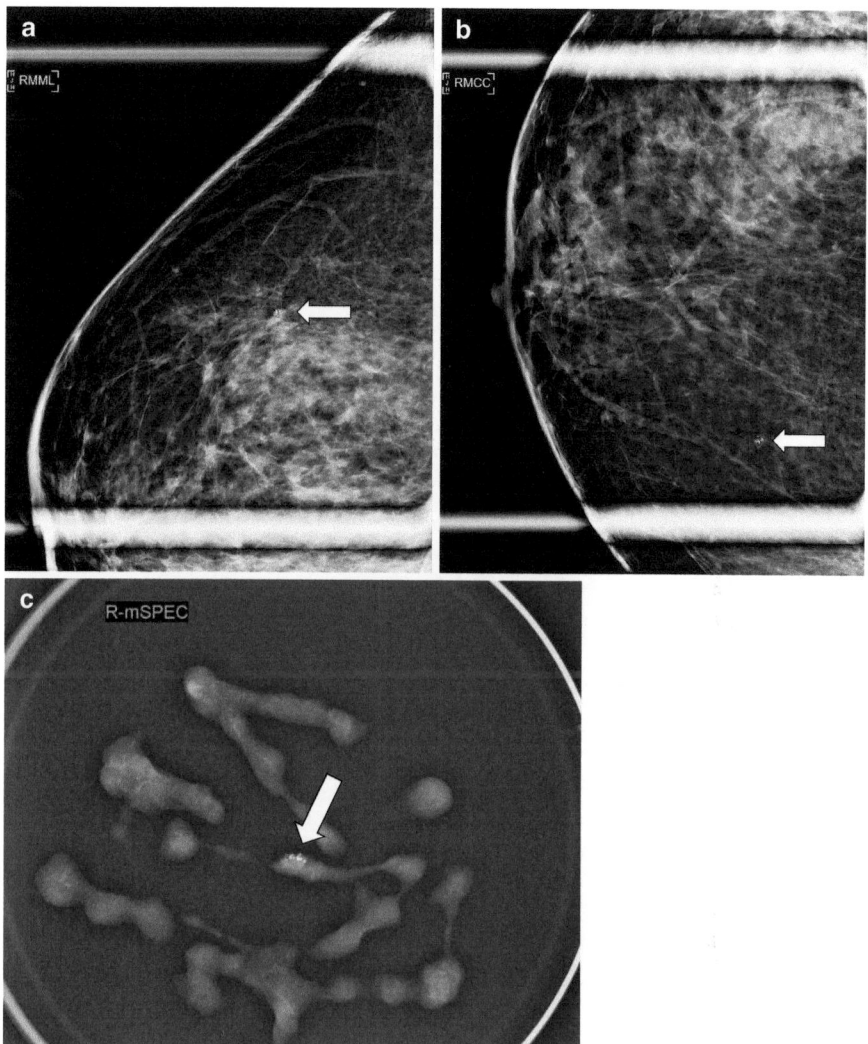

Fig. 6.7 Unexpected high-risk lesion as an incidental finding at biopsy. Clinical: new, grouped coarse heterogeneous calcifications in the right breast. BI-RADS 4A. Tissue diagnosis: ALH, microcalcifications present in stromal fibrosis. Targeted calcifications were not associated with ALH. Recommended for surgical excision. (**a** and **b**) Compression magnification ML and CC view. Grouped coarse microcalcifications in right breast upper inner quadrant, middle depth, at about 1 o'clock. New since prior exam 1 year ago. (**c**) Sample radiograph. Targeted calcifications are seen within a single sample in the image center (white arrow). Multiple other samples contain no calcifications. (**d**) Post-biopsy mammogram in CC projection. Air bubble is seen at the biopsy site. Biopsy marker clip (gray arrowhead) is seen 10 mm medial and slightly posterior to residual calcifications (white arrow). Clip distance from the targeted lesion should be measured in both projections (ML image not shown), calipers with measurements saved in PACS and values recorded in the biopsy report. When patient presents for preoperative needle localization, clip migration has to be taken into account. In this case, residual calcifications, not the marker clip, were targeted at needle localization

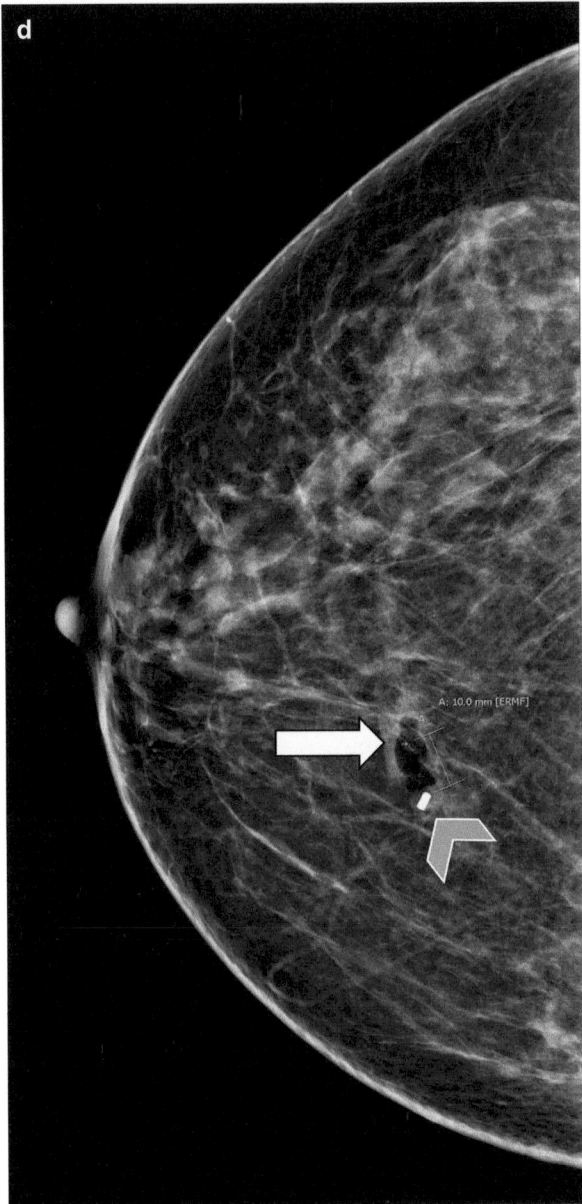

Fig. 6.7 (continued)

For example, grouped amorphous calcifications can be seen in FA, FCC, and DCIS. Pathological diagnosis is FA, which matches our differential diagnosis. That would be concordant benign pathology result, based on the first condition. Next comes the question: Is our suspicion low enough? Amorphous calcifications as a class are categorized as BI-RADS 4B lesion (10% < likelihood of malignancy <= 50%). If there were other groups of amorphous calcifications present in the same and contralateral breast, our suspicion would have been at the lower end of 4B range, or we would even assess them as BI-RADS 4A. In that case we would accept FA as concordant pathology result and recommend imaging follow-up in 1 year.

Benign pathology results for lesions categorized as BI-RADS 5 (likelihood of malignancy 95% and more) are clearly discordant, since benign pathology cannot explain imaging appearance assessed as highly suggestive of malignancy. Unless there was an obvious error, for example, a wrong lesion was sampled, or the biopsy needle completely missed the target, surgical excision will be recommended.

On the other end of spectrum, benign or probably benign lesions are sometimes sampled due to patient's preference and not because of our recommendation. Anything but matching benign pathology results would come as a surprise in these cases. Such matching benign results will be rendered concordant with recommendation for routine annual imaging follow-up. In young patients, under age of 40, who presented with palpable mass categorized as BI-RADS 3, with pathological diagnosis of FA, clinical follow-up is recommended, sometimes with ultrasound surveillance – depending on particular case. Most surgeons will consider excision if it grows in subsequent months or years. In case it was sizeable to start with, usually over 3 cm in maximum dimension, surgical excision might be considered from the start, regardless of concordant benign pathological diagnosis.

Here is the place to say few words about conveying BI-RADS 3 results to a patient, since many patients can potentially end up with unnecessary biopsy of probably benign lesion due to poor communication.

Probably benign result is best communicated by physician, usually a trainee in academic settings, but an experienced nurse can easily be trained to take over this task in busy practice. Few points should be clearly explained at the end of diagnostic encounter, before patient leaves the facility:

1. Based on imaging appearance and clinical data, we think that the lesion in question is probably benign and has low likelihood of malignancy, up to 2%. That means that, on average, one or two among a hundred patients with BI-RADS 3 lesion in fact have cancer.
2. There are two management options: short-term imaging follow-up and biopsy.

Both options should be described in sufficient detail, as follows:

(a) Short-term follow-up imaging is done to assess the lesion for changes over time. Two years stability is considered as a proof of benignity. Exact follow-up imaging strategy should be disclosed. It will depend on particular case, but for probably benign mass seen on baseline mammography and on targeted ultrasound, for example, it could be as follows: targeted ultrasound in 6 months, followed by bilateral mammography and targeted ultrasound in 12 months and again in 24 months, to confirm lesion's benign nature.

Important notes:

- If the lesion's appearance on follow-up imaging changes to worse at any point, or if palpable lesion grows, biopsy will be recommended.
- If the lesion gets smaller or is no longer seen on follow-up imaging, regular screening will resume.

(b) Biopsy is a minimally invasive procedure where small tissue samples are obtained and examined under the microscope. It is done in local anesthesia under imaging guidance using the biopsy needle. It is an accurate procedure with low risk of complications. It usually leaves minimal or no scar. Patient comes to breast imaging suite for the biopsy and goes home after the procedure.

3. We recommend follow-up imaging, but patient makes the choice.

For some patients "2% and less" chance for malignancy is an unacceptably high probability, and they might want sampling. Patient's understanding of her findings will depend on many socioeconomic factors. Radiologist should ensure that the patient or her legal representative understands medical terms like "benign" and "malignant" and has no misconceptions about the imaging-guided biopsy and pathologic entity in question. Patient might perceive cancer as incurable disease, basically a death sentence. It is our duty to acknowledge patient's beliefs, to convey the results and recommendations in layman's terms, and to address patient's concerns.

Some patients will simply go with radiologist's recommendation, but it is important to underline that there is a risk, however small, and that the choice is hers. This might be perceived as unfair, since patients in general lack the knowledge needed to reach informed decision. It often comes to answering patient's question: "What would you recommend if I was your family member?"

There will be cases when patient needs more time to decide. She should then be provided with direct phone number to communicate her decision to us at later time.

All relevant details of this encounter should be documented in radiology report. Trainees must be made aware of these particularities, since they are clinically important and also serve as a solid evidence for optimal patient care in malpractice cases.

For BI-RADS 4 assessment category, concordance assessment and management recommendations will vary the most. When we use subcategories, things become clearer.

BI-RADS 4A lesions (2% < likelihood of malignancy ≤10%) with matching benign pathology results are almost always rendered concordant, resulting in recommendation for imaging follow-up: routine annual or short term, depending on suspicion level and clinical circumstances.

Majority of BI-RADS 4C lesions (50% < likelihood of malignancy <95%) with matching benign pathology results will be recommended for surgical excision regardless, simply because our level of suspicion is too high.

BI-RADS 4B subcategory (10% < likelihood of malignancy ≤50%) is the least consistent one, where benign pathology results can be both accepted or rejected. In these cases, we decide about management based on all available information, not only the lesion's imaging appearance. BI-RADS Atlas does not and cannot offer precise management recommendations. Clinical thinking – combining patient's history, clinical presentation, imaging findings, and pathological diagnosis – should be the major force guiding our decision in all cases. About 1/4 of cases rendered discordant at Rad-Path correlation are found to be malignant on surgical excision, justifying this approach [4, 22, 23].

High-Risk Lesions

There is one group of pathologic entities which deserve particular attention in Rad-Path correlation. These entities have potential to further complicate our management decisions. For all practical purposes, however, at Rad-Path correlation, they are treated almost as if they were malignant [24–27]. These are high-risk lesions (HRL). When found on biopsy, they indicate increased risk for future breast cancer development. HRL can be precursor lesion, with increased risk for cancer development in ipsilateral breast, or is often seen in association with malignancy, indicating increased risk for breast cancer in both breasts.

HRL include:

- ADH
- Lobular neoplasia: LCIS, ALH
- FEA
- Radial scar/complex sclerosing lesion
- Papillary lesions

Relative risk (RR) for subsequent development of breast cancer is increased in patients with HRL [28, 29]. Reported RR estimates vary slightly but are in the range of 4–10 times of that in general population: LCIS carries RR of up to 10x, while ADH and ALH have RR of 4x for cancer development in both breasts. RR is further increased in patients with positive family history. While risk-reduction strategies and interventions, like anti-estrogen therapy, can be employed in these patients [30], there is no general consensus in management of HRL.

Intraductal epithelial proliferation in the breast is currently classified in three groups: usual ductal hyperplasia (UDH), ADH, and DCIS [31]. UDH is a benign proliferative entity, with no atypical cells. In both ADH and DCIS, there are cells with nuclear atypia. The difference between the two can be quantitative: ADH exists when atypical proliferation is seen in up to two ducts, while three or more contiguous ducts involved or total size over 2 mm satisfy the pathologic criteria for DCIS [26]. Differentiation between ADH and DCIS can be difficult for pathologists, as mentioned before. In fact, when ADH is found at imaging-guided biopsy, up to 1/4 of these lesions will be diagnosed as DCIS on subsequent surgical excision or even represent invasive carcinoma. In those cases, we are talking about histologic underestimation of disease: initial tissue diagnosis is upgraded at surgery, when the whole lesion is available for histological examination. Given the high upgrade rate, practically all cases of ADH at imaging-guided biopsy are recommended for surgical excision [4, 25, 26].

Histologic underestimation has been reported with other pathologic entities, as well: FEA, ALH, LCIS, and radial scar (RS), as well as DCIS, can all be upgraded to invasive carcinoma at surgical excision [4, 25, 26, 32]. There is wide variation in reported upgrade rates of HRL. In average, they are highest for ADH and LCIS but are well above 2% threshold for all these lesions, leading to recommendation for surgical excision in majority of cases [25].

RS, also called complex sclerosing lesion (CSL) when larger than 1 cm in size, can be associated with atypia, in situ, or invasive cancer. RS presents as architectural distortion and can mimic tubular carcinoma, both radiologically and pathologically. Unless incidental, with no imaging correlate, and microscopic in size, surgical excision is recommended [1, 25].

Asymptomatic solitary intraductal papilloma without atypia, according to newer studies, can be followed by imaging since the upgrade rate on surgical excision is about 2% [33–35]. If there is atypia or in situ carcinoma found within the papillary lesion, surgical excision is recommended. In practice, pathologist might recommend surgical excision due to incomplete sampling of papilloma, when they estimate that less than 50% of the lesion is present in sample.

Authors are trying to identify subgroups of HRL which might be safe to follow up after they were diagnosed on tissue sampling. There are reports of low upgrade rates, around 2%, for cases of pure FEA and pure LCIS presenting as suspicious calcifications, where all the calcifications were removed at biopsy [36–38]. Investigative work in this regard is hampered with low incidence of these lesions resulting in small series, simultaneous presence of various HRL in the samples and variable thresholds in pathology reporting [25].

There are other rare pathologic entities which are considered controversial and are routinely recommended for surgical excision after being found on sampling. They include phyllodes tumors, mucocele-like lesions with atypia, granular-cell tumors, and desmoid tumors [26, 39]. Some benign lesions can be recommended for excision, based on their growth documented on imaging over time and overall size. Those include complex FA and pseudoangiomatous stromal hyperplasia (PASH).

Better understanding of breast disease processes will inevitably lead to changes in management recommendations in the future. For some patients, watchful waiting might represent better strategy than surgical excision [40].

In conclusion, Rad-Path correlation is the final step in diagnostic process, where clinical management recommendation is made. One should strive to make this process as robust as possible, thus providing the optimal patient care.

References

1. Bassett LW, Mahoney MC, Apple SK. Interventional breast imaging: current procedures and assessing for concordance with pathology. Radiol Clin N Am. 2007;45(5):881–94.
2. Youk JH, Kim EK, Kim MJ, Ko KH, Kwak JY, Son EJ, Choi J, Kang HY. Concordant or discordant? Imaging-pathology correlation in a sonography-guided core needle biopsy of a breast lesion. Korean J Radiol. 2011;12(2):232–40.
3. D'Orsi CJ, Sickles EA, Mendelson EB, Morris EA, et al. ACR BI-RADS® atlas, breast imaging reporting and data system. Reston: American College of Radiology; 2013.
4. Liberman L. Percutaneous image-guided core breast biopsy. Radiol Clin N Am. 2002;40:483–50.
5. Bagnall MJ, Evans AJ, Wilson AR, Burrell H, Pinder SE, Ellis IO. When have mammographic calcifications been adequately sampled at needle core biopsy? Clin Radiol. 2000;55(7):548–53.
6. Eby PR, Ochsner JE, DeMartini WB, Allison KH, Peacock S, Lehman CD. Frequency and upgrade rates of atypical ductal hyperplasia diagnosed at stereotactic vacuum-assisted breast biopsy: 9-versus 11-gauge. AJR Am J Roentgenol. 2009;192(1):229–34.
7. Lourenco AP, Mainiero MB, Lazarus E, Giri D, Schepps B. Stereotactic breast biopsy: comparison of histologic underestimation rates with 11- and 9-gauge vacuum-assisted breast biopsy. AJR Am J Roentgenol. 2007;189(5):W275–9.
8. Brem RF, Schoonjans JM, Goodman SN, Nolten A, Askin FB, Gatewood OM. Nonpalpable breast cancer: percutaneous diagnosis with 11- and 8-gauge stereotactic vacuum-assisted biopsy devices. Radiology. 2001;219(3):793–6.
9. Ruggirello I, Nori J, Desideri I, Saieva C, Giannotti E, Bicchierai G, De Benedetto D, Francolini G, Bianchi S, Vezzosi V, Sanchez L, Susini T, Orzalesi L, Meattini I, Livi L, Miele V. Stereotactic vacuum-assisted breast biopsy: comparison between 11- and 8-gauge needles. Eur J Surg Oncol. 2017;43(12):2257–60.
10. Parikh J, Tickman R. Image-guided tissue sampling: where radiology meets pathology. Breast J. 2005;11(6):403–9.
11. Sorace J, Aberle DR, Elimam D, Lawvere S, Tawfik O, Wallace WD. Integrating pathology and radiology disciplines: an emerging opportunity? BMC Med. 2012;10:100.
12. Nomenclature of antigen names. http://cvc.dfci.harvard.edu/cvccgi/tadb/nomenclature.pl. Accessed on 31 Oct 2018
13. Allison KH, Rendi MH, Peacock S, Morgan T, Elmore JG, Weaver DL. Histological features associated with diagnostic agreement in atypical ductal hyperplasia of the breast: illustrative cases from the B-path study. Histopathology. 2016;69(6):1028–46.
14. Jain RK, Mehta R, Dimitrov R, Larsson LG, Musto PM, Hodges KB, Ulbright TM, Hattab EM, Agaram N, Idrees MT, Badve S. Atypical ductal hyperplasia: interobserver and intraobserver variability. Mod Pathol. 2011;24(7):917–23. https://doi.org/10.1038/modpathol.2011.66. Epub 2011 Apr 29.
15. Tozbikian G, Brogi E, Vallejo CE, Giri D, Murray M, Catalano J, Olcese C, Van Zee KJ, Wen HY. Atypical ductal hyperplasia bordering on ductal carcinoma in situ. Int J Surg Pathol. 2017;25(2):100–7.
16. Samples LS, Rendi MH, Frederick PD, Allison KH, Nelson HD, Morgan TR, Weaver DL, Elmore JG. Surgical implications and variability in the use of the flat epithelial atypia diagnosis on breast biopsy specimens. Breast. 2017;34:34–43.

17. Lesslie MD, Parikh JR. Multidisciplinary tumor boards: an opportunity for radiologists to demonstrate value. Acad Radiol. 2017;24(1):107–10.
18. Krishnamurthy S, Bevers T, Kuerer HM, Smith B, Yang WT. AJR paradigm shifts in breast care delivery: impact of imaging in a multidisciplinary environment. AJR Am J Roentgenol. 2017;208(2):248–55.
19. Foster TJ, Bouchard-Fortier A, Olivotto IA, Quan ML. Effect of multidisciplinary case conferences on physician decision making: breast diagnostic rounds. Cureus. 2016;8(11):e895.
20. Esserman LE, Cura MA, DaCosta D. Recognizing pitfalls in early and late migration of clip markers after imaging-guided directional vacuum-assisted biopsy. Radiographics. 2004;24(1):147–56.
21. Sohn YM, Yoon JH, Kim EK, Moon HJ, Kim MJ. Percutaneous ultrasound-guided vacuum-assisted removal versus surgery for breast lesions showing imaging-histology discordance after ultrasound-guided core-needle biopsy. Korean J Radiol. 2014;15(6):697–703.
22. Son EJ, Kim EK, Youk JH, Kim MJ, Kwak JY, Choi SH. Imaging-histologic discordance after sonographically guided percutaneous breast biopsy: a prospective observational study. Ultrasound Med Biol. 2011;37(11):1771–8.
23. Soyder A, Taşkin F, Ozbas S. Imaging-histological discordance after sonographically guided percutaneous breast core biopsy. Breast Care. 2015;10(1):33–7.
24. Berg WA. Image-guided breast biopsy and management of high-risk lesions. Radiol Clin N Am. 2004;42:935–46.
25. Mooney KL, Bassett LW, Apple SK. Upgrade rates of high-risk breast lesions diagnosed on core needle biopsy: a single-institution experience and literature review. Mod Pathol. 2016;29(12):1471–84.
26. Neal L, Sandhu NP, Hieken TJ, Glazebrook KN, Mac Bride MB, Dilaveri CA, Wahner-Roedler DL, Ghosh K, Visscher DW. Diagnosis and management of benign, atypical, and indeterminate breast lesions detected on core needle biopsy. Mayo Clin Proc. 2014;89(4):536–47.
27. Javitt MC. Diagnosis and management of high-risk breast lesions: Aristotle's dilemma. Am J Roentgenol. 2012;198:246–8.
28. Hartmann LC, Sellers TA, Frost MH, Lingle WL, Degnim AC, Ghosh K, Vierkant RA, Maloney SD, Pankratz VS, Hillman DW, Suman VJ, Johnson J, Blake C, Tlsty T, Vachon CM, Melton LJ, Visscher DW. Benign breast disease and the risk of breast cancer. N Engl J Med. 2005;353(3):229–37.
29. London SJ, Connolly JL, Schnitt SJ, Colditz GA. A prospective study of benign breast disease and the risk of breast cancer. JAMA. 1992;267(7):941–4.
30. Brewster AM, Thomas P, Brown P, Coyne R, Yan Y, Checka C, Middleton L, Do KA, Bevers T. A system-level approach to improve the uptake of anti-estrogen preventive therapy among women with atypical hyperplasia and lobular cancer in situ. Cancer Prev Res. 2018;11:295–302.
31. Purcell CA, Norris HJ. Intraductal proliferations of the breast: a review of histologic criteria for atypical intraductal hyperplasia and ductal carcinoma in situ, including apocrine and papillary lesions. Ann Diagn Pathol. 1998;2(2):135–45.
32. Brennan ME, Turner RM, Ciatto S, Marinovich ML, French JR, Macaskill P, Houssami N. Ductal carcinoma in situ at core-needle biopsy: meta-analysis of underestimation and predictors of invasive breast cancer. Radiology. 2011;260(1):119–28.
33. Han SH, Kim M, Chung YR, Yun B, Jang M, Kim SM, Kang E, Kim EK, Park SY. Benign intraductal papilloma without atypia on core needle biopsy has a low rate of upgrading to malignancy after excision. J Breast Cancer. 2018;21(1):80–6.
34. Ko D, Kang E, Park SY, Kim SM, Jang M, Yun B, Chae S, Jang Y, Kim HJ, Kim SW, Kim EK. The management strategy of benign solitary intraductal papilloma on breast core biopsy. Clin Breast Cancer. 2017;17(5):367–72.
35. Pareja F, Corben AD, Brennan SB, Murray MP, Bowser ZL, Jakate K, Sebastiano C, Morrow M, Morris EA, Brogi E. Breast intraductal papillomas without atypia in radiologic-pathologic concordant core-needle biopsies: rate of upgrade to carcinoma at excision. Cancer. 2016;122(18):2819–27.

36. Calhoun BC, Sobel A, White RL, Gromet M, Flippo T, Sarantou T, Livasy CA. Management of flat epithelial atypia on breast core biopsy may be individualized based on correlation with imaging studies. Mod Pathol. 2015;28(5):670–6.
37. Lamb LR, Bahl M, Gadd MA, Lehman CD. Flat epithelial atypia: upgrade rates and risk-stratification approach to support informed decision making. J Am Coll Surg. 2017;225(6):696–701.
38. Susnik B, Day D, Abeln E, Bowman T, Krueger J, Swenson KK, Tsai ML, Bretzke ML, Lillemoe TJ. Surgical outcomes of lobular neoplasia diagnosed in core biopsy: prospective study of 316 cases. Clin Breast Cancer. 2016;16(6):507–13.
39. Ha SM, Cha JH, Shin HJ, Chae EY, Choi WJ, Kim HH. Mucocelelike lesions in the breast: radiologic and clinicopathologic correlations with upgrade rate. AJR Am J Roentgenol. 2018;210(6):1386–94.
40. A trial comparing surgery with active monitoring for low risk DCIS (LORIS). https://www.cancerresearchuk.org/about-cancer/find-a-clinical-trial/a-trial-comparing-surgery-with-active-monitoring-for-low-risk-dcis-loris. Accessed 31 Oct 2018.

Index